Clinical
Governance in
HEALTH CARE
PRACTICE

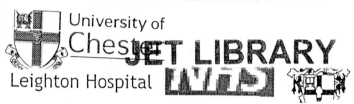

University of
Chester
Leighton Hospital

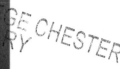

For Butterworth-Heinemann:

Commissioning Editor: Susan Young
Development Editor: Catherine Jackson
Project Manager: Morven Dean
Design: George Ajayi

Clinical Governance in HEALTH CARE PRACTICE

SECOND EDITION

Thoreya Swage MBBS(Lond) MA(Oxon)
Visiting Fellow, University of Reading
Consultant in Healthcare Management

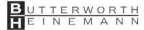

EDINBURGH LONDON NEW YORK PHILADELPHIA
ST LOUIS SYDNEY TORONTO 2003

BUTTERWORTH-HEINEMANN
An imprint of Elsevier Science Limited

First edition 2000
Reprinted 2000, 2001 (twice)

ISBN 0 7506 5681 6

British Library Cataloguing in Publication Data
A catalogue record for this book is available from the British Library

Library of Congress Cataloging in Publication Data
A catalog record for this book is available from the Library of Congress

Note
Medical knowledge is constantly changing. Standard safety precautions must be followed, but as new research and clinical experience broaden our knowledge, changes in treatment and drug therapy may become necessary or appropriate. Readers are advised to check the most current product information provided by the manufacturer of each drug to be administered to verify the recommended dose, the method and duration of administration, and contraindications. It is the responsibility of the practitioner, relying on experience and knowledge of the patient, to determine dosages and the best treatment for each individual patient. Neither the Publisher nor the author assumes any liability for any injury and/or damage to persons or property arising from this publication.

The Publisher

ELSEVIER
SCIENCE

your source for books,
journals and multimedia
in the health sciences

www.elsevierhealth.com

The
publisher's
policy is to use
**paper manufactured
from sustainable forests**

Printed in China

Contents

Acknowledgements

I would like to thank the following who helped to make the second edition of my book possible in various ways:

Nicci Iacovou, who provided helpful information on some of the management processes and detailed comments on the manuscript; Christopher Newdick of Reading University who looked over Chapter 10; Mary Dunne of Frimley Park Hospital and Maureen Swage.

I would also like to thank the following for permission to reproduce their material in the second edition of this book:

Her Majesty's Stationery Office (Crown copyright material is reproduced with permission of the Controller of Her Majesty's Stationery Office); The Nursing and Midwifery Council; Tangent Medical Education; The AGREE Collaboration (www.agreecollaboration.org) and Croner.CCH Group Ltd.

Finally I would like to thank my family, Ben, Zahra and Fayrouz for their patience, tolerance, encouragement and support during the second round of writing of the book.

Foreword

Since the first edition of the book was published in 2000, there have been many developments in the sphere of clinical governance which are worthy of inclusion.

Although the principles of clinical governance have remained the same, much of the updating for the second edition is around the policy, strategy and legal and ethical changes that have occurred since clinical governance was first proposed in 1997.

The book otherwise retains the original subject headings and chapters, examples of aspects of clinical governance to illustrate certain points and the toolkit at the end for the reader to use as a resource. This edition, however, has been augmented with a list of some of the useful, relevant websites referred to in the text.

Although the structures and functions of the bodies that implement clinical governance do change, the book still aims to provide some of the essential principles upon which the quality of health care can improve and develop.

Dr Thoreya Swage
October 2003

1

Introduction – Clinical governance and the wider quality agenda

Imagine the following scenarios:

- A psychiatric nurse allows a sectioned mental health patient who has been on one-to-one care to go out 'round the corner' to buy some cigarettes. The patient goes 'absent without leave' and is found by the police in a ditch having overdosed on drugs.
- A senior registrar continues to perform major surgery on patients, but he has not revealed to the occupational health physicians that he is HIV positive because he is afraid of losing his job.
- An acute hospital trust board receives reports of poor outcomes on paediatric cardiac surgery; however, nothing is followed up.
- The archaic sewage system of an old hospital building overflows and causes a great risk of infection and hygiene to patients on the affected wards.
- An experienced community midwife attempts to deliver a woman in her home, and her baby has an awkward presentation. The attempt is unsuccessful; the woman is rushed as an emergency to hospital and the baby is born with a fractured clavicle.
- A consultant physician continues to prescribe expensive medicines for respiratory conditions when there is no robust evidence to support their use in achieving better outcomes compared to older, cheaper alternatives.
- A complaint is made by the relatives of a stroke patient who died unexpectedly following a fall from a hospital bed. They claim that the patient was given inadequate care because cot sides were not erected on the bed.

- A female GP is called out at two o'clock in the morning to assess a middle-aged man who is acting strangely. His lodgings are situated in a run-down estate that is well known for drug dealing activities.

Any clinician or manager working in health care will recognise these types of scenarios, some of which are, incidentally, taken from real life. They will have occurred in one form or another in a number of health care settings. Several questions arise – what should be done when faced with these situations? Is the action appropriate and effective, and are lessons learnt from these events so that they do not recur? Is there an overall responsibility for co-ordinating these different quality areas? Is there any accountability within the organisation for things going wrong, and for an improvement programme to address the issues raised? Is quality a priority?

In the White Paper *The New NHS, Modern, Dependable,*[1] the recently elected Labour government declared in 1997 that 'The new NHS will have quality at its heart'. This marked the beginning of a 10-year quality improvement programme for the National Health Service, which aimed to 'guarantee fair access and high quality to patients wherever they live'.[2]

This declaration was triggered by a number of factors that were perceived to have undermined public confidence in the National Health Service. These included the capacity of the service to keep up with the accelerating advances in medical technology and treatments, the greater demands by the general public, changes in working patterns and family life, and the ageing population. In addition, there have been claims of inequalities in access to health care based on where people live, the so called 'postcode prescribing' – for example, the availability of infertility treatment, or of new drugs such as interferon for multiple sclerosis, or differential waiting times for outpatients and operations. Some variations are described in the box below. Finally, a series of lapses in the quality of care, which made headline news, such as the failures of cervical cancer

---

Some variations in the delivery of health care across the UK[1]

- In Manchester, the death rate from coronary heart disease in people aged less than 65 is nearly three times higher than in West Surrey.
- The number of hip replacements in people aged over 65 varies from 10 to 51 per 10 000 of the population.
- The number of people seen in outpatients within 13 weeks of a written GP referral varies from 71% to 98%.
- The percentage of drugs prescribed generically varies from below 50% to almost 70%.

screening in Kent and Canterbury Hospital[3] and similarly of breast cancer screening in Exeter, had prompted doubts about overall standards of care.

In the White Paper, *A First Class Service*,[2] the agenda for quality was set, connecting the clinical judgement of individual practitioners with clear agreed national standards for health care.

In this document, three main components for ensuring high quality care were outlined:

● The setting of clear standards – including the role of the National Institute for Clinical Excellence (England and Wales), the Clinical Standards Board for Scotland (Scotland), the Scottish Inter-Collegiate Guidelines Network (Scotland) and the National Service Frameworks (England).
● The delivery of those standards locally, in a consistent manner and with the involvement of the general public – through clinical governance, life-long learning and professional self-regulation.
● Standards that are monitored – via the Commission for Health Improvement* (England and Wales), the Clinical Standards Board for Scotland (Scotland), the National Patient Safety Agency (England), the National Performance Frameworks and the National Patient and User Surveys.

WHAT IS CLINICAL GOVERNANCE?

Although in the past it has been difficult to produce a universally accepted definition of clinical quality, the government has, for the first time, attempted to do this by the introduction of the idea of clinical governance. This builds on an idea previously put forward by the World Health Organisation[4] where quality is described as the following four elements:

● Professional management (technical quality)
● Resource use (efficiency)
● Risk management (including the risk of injury or illness associated from the service provided)
● Satisfaction of patients with the service provided.

Since 1 April 1999, all National Health Service bodies in the United Kingdom have had the new statutory duty of clinical governance placed

---

Footnote

* At the time of writing, subject to primary legislation, the Commission for Health Improvement will be superceded by a new body called the Commission for Healthcare Audit and Inspection.

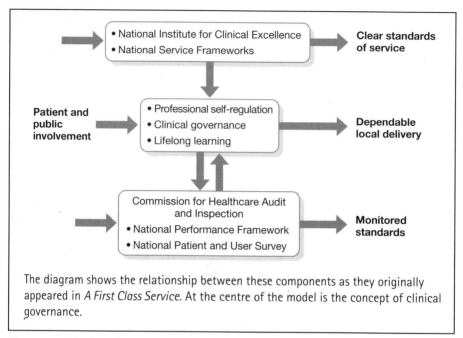

The diagram shows the relationship between these components as they originally appeared in *A First Class Service*. At the centre of the model is the concept of clinical governance.

Figure 1.1 Setting, delivering, monitoring standards – from *A First Class Service*[2]

upon them. For the first time since the inception of the NHS in 1948, accountability for the quality of clinical care delivered by clinicians became an important requirement throughout the organisation, the responsibility finally resting with the Chief Executive. The same standards also apply to the private sector.

This responsibility of clinical governance involves guaranteeing quality through a number of processes, many of which are currently in use and should be familiar to any clinician or manager. They include clinical effectiveness, clinical risk management, complaints, professional development, outcomes of care and good quality clinical data. This duty is equal to the other statutory responsibility of NHS organisations, which is of financial probity, accountability and ensuring value for public money on behalf of the taxpayer. However, unlike in the past, when the focus was on how many more patients could be treated each year, or whether waiting times were on target or not, the quality of clinical care no longer occupies the 'second best' position in board-level discussions.

The White Paper, *The New NHS, Modern, Dependable* makes it very clear that clinical governance places a duty on all health professionals, clinicians and managers alike, to ensure that the level of clinical service they deliver to patients is 'satisfactory, consistent and responsive'.

This shift in focus from a purely financial perspective recognises the essential role of clinicians in quality processes and appropriately places the responsibility for developing and maintaining clinical standards within their local NHS organisations on their shoulders. The expertise of nurses, doctors and other clinical professionals is pivotal in helping their organisations to achieve this goal.

So what is clinical governance? What does this mean in reality for busy clinicians? Essentially, clinical governance provides an umbrella under which all aspects of quality can be gathered and continuously monitored. It is about providing or not providing the carrots to clinicians, rather than the sticks to improve health care, and this also has to be led by clinicians.

> The White Paper, *A First Class Service*, defines clinical governance as:
> 'A framework through which NHS organisations are accountable for continuously improving the quality of their services and safeguarding high standards of care by creating an environment in which clinical care will flourish'.[2]

Clinical governance was initially developed for NHS trusts, and comprises the following processes:[2]

1. Clear lines of responsibility and accountability for the overall quality of clinical care:

- The NHS trust Chief Executive carries ultimate responsibility for the quality of services provided by the trust
- A designated senior clinician, ideally at board level, is responsible for ensuring that systems of clinical governance are in place and monitoring their continued effectiveness
- There are formal arrangements for NHS trust boards to discharge their responsibilities for clinical quality, for example, perhaps through a clinical governance committee
- Regular reports should be made to the trust board on the quality of clinical care, and given the same importance as monthly financial reports
- An annual report on clinical governance should be produced, which is open to public scrutiny.

2. A comprehensive programme of quality improvement activities, including:

- Full participation by all hospital doctors in audit programmes, including specialty and sub-specialty national external audit programmes endorsed by the Commission for Health Improvement (CHI)

- Full participation in the current four National Confidential Enquiries
  - National Confidential Enquiry into Perioperative Deaths (NCEPOD)
  - Confidential Enquiry into Stillbirths and Deaths in Infancy (CESDI)
  - Confidential Enquiry into Maternal Deaths (CEMD)
  - Confidential Inquiry into Suicide and Homicide by People with Mental Illness (CISH)
- Evidence-based practice that is supported and routinely applied in everyday practice
- Ensuring the clinical standards of National Service Frameworks and National Institute for Clinical Excellence recommendations are implemented
- Workforce planning and development (i.e. recruitment and retention of an appropriately trained workforce) is fully integrated within the NHS trust's service planning
- Continuing professional development: programmes aimed at meeting the development needs of individual health professionals and the service needs of the organisation are in place and supported locally and regularly monitored
- Appropriate safeguards to govern access to and storage of confidential patient information as recommended by the Caldicott Report[5] on the review of patient-identifiable information
- Effective monitoring of clinical care with high quality systems for clinical record keeping and the collection of relevant information
- Processes for assuring the quality of clinical care are in place and integrated with the quality programme for the organisation as a whole.

3. Clear policies aimed at managing risk:

- Controls assurance, which promotes self-assessment to identify and manage risks
- Clinical risk systematically assessed with programmes in place to reduce risk.

4. Procedures for all professional groups to identify and remedy poor performance:

- Critical incident reporting to ensure that adverse incidents are identified and openly investigated, and that lessons are learned and promptly applied
- Complaints procedures, accessible to patients and their families and fair to staff, so that lessons are learned and the recurrence of similar problems avoided

- Professional performance procedures which take effect at an early stage before patients are harmed, and which help individuals to improve their performance, whenever possible, in place and understood by all staff
- Staff supported in their duty to report any concerns about colleagues' professional conduct and performance, with clear statements from the board on what is expected of them. Clear procedures for reporting concerns so that early action can be taken to support the individual and remedy the situation.

Clinical governance has been further refined into the 'seven pillars' which are:[6]

- Clinical effectiveness – ensuring that interventions and treatments are based on the best available research evidence.
- Risk management – reducing the potential for unwanted outcomes when treating patients, including learning from mistakes.
- Research and development – carrying out research, critically appraising papers and interpreting the evidence into useable form for busy health care professionals (e.g. guidelines).

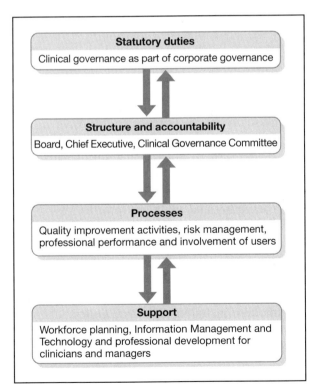

Figure 1.2 The main components of clinical governance

- Use of the workforce – ensuring that planning of the numbers and types of health care professionals is in line with the requirements of the health service
- Training and education – ensuring that health care professionals are appropriately trained for the tasks they are required to undertake.
- Use of information technology – ensuring that health care professionals have easy access to the research evidence and best practice examples in the country and abroad.
- Patient/user feedback – ensuring that quality is patient/user centred.

This book aims to take the reader through the different elements of clinical governance outlined above and the following chapters demonstrate the links between each of the processes that contribute to the improvement of the quality of health care. It has been recognised that clinical governance is an evolving process, and that not all the answers are immediately obvious or available; however, the book aims to provide an introduction to the concept by highlighting areas of importance through some examples of local implementation and by raising issues for further consideration.

Figure 1.2 illustrates the main components of clinical governance. These will be expanded further in the ensuing chapters.

Issues for further consideration

- What does clinical governance mean to you and your organisation?
- What opportunities and threats are presented by clinical governance?

First responses to new ideas are usually reactive and often defensive; clinical governance is no exception. The fears of restricted clinical freedom, policing and criticism of clinical expertise are commonplace. However, the essence of clinical governance is that this is an opportunity for clinicians to take the lead in the delivery of health care, to demonstrate how that can be done effectively, to learn from each other and share best practice in a structured way. Addressing quality issues can highlight true need and generate a debate on how limited resources can best be used. Clinical governance also provides the opportunity for individual health care professionals to fulfil their obligations concerning continued development and updating which, in the past, have been difficult to pursue. Indeed, this is an area that the professional bodies (including the Royal College of Nursing, the General Medical Council, the Royal Colleges, etc.) have been actively promoting, whilst highlighting poor access to further training and development.

Where does clinical governance sit with other NHS policies?

It is intended that clinical governance is very much integrated with other strategies guiding the NHS and that it does not operate in isolation of, or work antagonistically against, other priorities.

On a local level this co-ordination is achieved through a 3-year planning framework for the development of local services called the Local Delivery Plan (LDP).[7] The LDP covers a Strategic Health Authority area and is based on Primary Care Trust (PCT) level plans. The plans are developed in partnership with other bodies including social services and acute trusts. The clinical governance programme must link in with the LDP. By doing this, the commissioning of effective evidence-based care by PCTs is strengthened and becomes a major component of the service level agreements (or contracts) for the delivery of care within trusts. Similarly, the monitoring of the delivery of care through *The NHS Performance Assessment Framework*[8] reinforces the implementation of the quality agenda by looking at outcomes of care. The inter-relationships between the different NHS policies and priorities are illustrated in Figure 1.3.

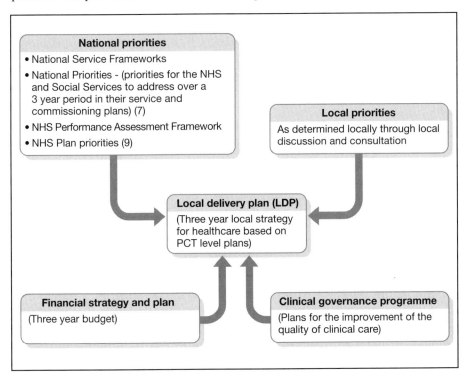

Figure 1.3 The inter-relationship between the different NHS policies and priorities. From *The NHS Performance Assessment Framework*[8]

Clearly it is not possible to have a plan to cover all the topics requiring further development in the clinical governance programme of an NHS organisation in 3 years. The clinical governance programme therefore is guided by the priorities identified in *The NHS Plan*, a document published in 2000, that sets out the government's plan for modernisation of the NHS.[9]

The aim is to provide a focus for developing and improving health care delivery in key health areas. By addressing clinical governance issues in coronary heart disease, for example, this will lead to better information on evidence-based commissioning and appropriate targeting of resources to more effective interventions.

THE SETTING AND MONITORING OF NATIONAL STANDARDS

There are variations in the availability and quality of health care to different patient groupings across the country. These have been highlighted by the publicised events mentioned earlier. The reports into the failures of cervical and breast cancer screening have common themes, such as poor training and communication within the teams, poor morale, little team working and deteriorating relations between technical staff, nurses, doctors and managers, all of which went unheeded over many years. It was repeated failure to address these specific areas which exposed the teams making mistakes to public scrutiny.

Issues for further consideration

● What impact has the publicising of 'health scares' had on you personally and on your team or organisation?

The exposure of health scares, particularly in the media, is detrimental not only to those concerned but also to people working in other organisations. The process can uncover a number of complex emotions and reactions. There may be worry about colleagues whose practice is of concern; irritation at uninformed media reports; an acknowledgement that the public needs to know about the issues; a highlighting of the difficulties in relationships between health professionals (e.g. doctors and nurses); and relief that the incident didn't happen here, or confidence that it couldn't happen here because good team working is in place.

The scenario of clinical care going astray is worsened by an ignorance of findings or a failure to learn lessons from the national confidential enquiries. The national confidential enquiries obtain information anonymously, on a voluntary basis, from all clinicians in four areas: deaths during or after surgery (initiated 1988); stillbirths and deaths in infancy (initiated 1991); maternal deaths (initiated 1951); and suicide and homicide by people with mental illness (initiated 1991). However, there seems to be little evidence of learning lessons from the findings or of using the information to improve care. For example, the Confidential Enquiry into Maternal Deaths (1994–5)[10] found that some maternal deaths were due to sub-standard care, misdiagnosed pulmonary embolism, ectopic pregnancy, puerperal sepsis, poor advice on how to wear a seat belt during pregnancy and failure to identify post-natal depression and domestic violence. These are areas that are familiar to those working in the field, and the issues have yet to be addressed in a systematic manner. With the development of clinical governance, participation will be a requirement for the relevant clinicians.

Clearly the setting of national standards is an important element in reducing these inequalities and concerns in the provision of health care. Such standards and the advice to support their implementation are delivered through the National Service Frameworks, the National Institute for Clinical Excellence, the Clinical Standards Board for Scotland and the Scottish Inter-Collegiate Guidelines Network.

The National Service Frameworks

The National Service Frameworks aim to ensure equity of access and standardisation of NHS care for patients, in whatever part of the country they happen to live. They are also a means whereby related policies are linked, reinforced and targeted towards a single direction – for example, the National Service Framework for coronary heart disease links together the Tobacco White Paper[11] and the National Priorities and Planning Framework.

The National Service Frameworks are steered by an external reference group for each subject, whose function is to advise the Department of Health on the whole system of care in the following areas:

- improving the quality of care and health outcomes using the best available evidence of clinical and cost effectiveness
- reducing undesirable variations in health care
- setting out the expectations of NHS care to the public and providers.

Implementation of the National Service Framework recommendations requires partnerships across a number of agencies, such as social services, the wider local authority (e.g. environmental health, housing and

- National Service Frameworks will set national standards and define service models for a specific service or care group.
- National Service Frameworks will bring together the best evidence of clinical and cost effectiveness with the views of service users to determine the best ways of providing particular services.[2]

education), the voluntary sector and other government departments. Each National Service Framework has the same terms of reference:[2]

- a definition of the scope and purpose of the Framework
- the evidence base, including:
  - a needs assessment
  - current performance in the NHS
  - clinical and cost effectiveness – the evidence to support this
  - identification of significant gaps and pressures in the service
- national standards and time scales for delivery
- an assessment of key interventions with associated costs
- work that has been commissioned to support implementation of the findings through
  - appropriate research and development projects, via the NHS research and development programme, which also includes Health Technology Assessments – for example, an assessment of new surgical techniques and new medical equipment
  - critical appraisal of current areas of good practice
  - the use of benchmarks against which to monitor implementation
  - a set of outcome indicators demonstrating effective care
- supporting programmes for implementation
  - workforce planning in all sectors of the NHS
  - recommended areas for further education and training
  - personal and organisational development
  - development of information management and technology
- a performance management framework for purchasers of health care to monitor the delivery of services.

Two subjects a year, on average, are tackled as part of a rolling programme for the National Service Frameworks. The criteria for selecting topics include:

- an area where there are inequalities in health, as outlined in *Saving Lives: Our Healthier Nation* and other related wider policies on social exclusion
- an important health issue, especially in terms of morbidity, mortality,

disability and use of resources
- an area that is of concern to the public
- an area where there is evidence of a gap between actual and accepted good practice, particularly if there are real opportunities for further development
- an area where the health care is provided in more than one setting (e.g. hospital, primary care or in the community) or by more than one type of organisation (e.g. both health and social services)
- an area where there is a need to reorganise or restructure local services to improve the delivery of care
- a problem that requires a different approach
- any relevant information arising from the Chief Medical Officer's Annual Report.

To date there have been the Calman-Hine National Service Frameworks for cancer services, coronary heart disease, mental health, older people and diabetes. Further topics include NSFs for children and for chronic neurological conditions.

The output of the National Service Frameworks includes a number of products; for example, standards relating to the content of care, systems and organisation of care, performance indicators, and various tools to support implementation of the recommendations.

The emerging findings from the National Service Framework for coronary heart disease (CHD) identified the following standards:[12]

- Population-wide approaches to health promotion and the prevention of coronary heart disease
- The identification and management of people at high risk of developing coronary heart disease, including cardiac rehabilitation
- The treatment of:
  - Chest pain (angina pectoris)
  - Heart attack (acute myocardial infarction)
  - Irregular heart beat (arrhythmia)
  - Heart failure.

In the final NSF,[13] these were developed further into the standards detailed in Table 1.1.

Implementation of these standards requires multiagency working across health and social care and other partners in the local community.

Table 1.1 NSF for CHD – Standards table[13]

Standards 1 & 2: Reducing heart disease in the population

1. The NHS and partner agencies should:
   develop, implement and monitor policies that reduce the prevalence of coronary risk factors in the population, and reduce inequalities in risks of developing heart disease.
2. The NHS and partner agencies should:
   contribute to a reduction in the prevalence of smoking in the local population.

Standards 3 & 4: Preventing CHD in high risk patients

3. General practitioners and primary care teams should:
   identify all people with established cardiovascular disease and offer them comprehensive advice and appropriate treatment to reduce their risks.
4. General practitioners and primary care teams should:
   identify all people at significant risk of cardiovascular disease but who have not developed symptoms and offer them appropriate advice and treatment to reduce their risks.

Standards 5, 6 & 7: Heart attack and other acute coronary syndromes

5. People with symptoms of a possible heart attack should:
   receive help from an individual equipped with and appropriately trained in the use of a defibrillator within 8 minutes of calling for help, to maximise the benefits of resuscitation should it be necessary.
6. People thought to be suffering from a heart attack should:
   be assessed professionally and, if indicated, receive aspirin. Thrombolysis should be given within 60 minutes of calling for professional help.
7. NHS Trusts should:
   put in place agreed protocols/systems of care so that people admitted to hospital with proven heart attack are appropriately assessed and offered treatments of proven clinical and cost effectiveness to reduce their risk of disability and death.

Standard 8: Stable angina

8. People with symptoms of angina or suspected angina should:
   receive appropriate investigation and treatment to relieve their pain and reduce their risk of coronary events.

Standards 9 & 10: Revascularisation

9. People with angina that is increasing in frequency or severity should:
   be referred to a cardiologist urgently or, for those at greatest risk, as an emergency.

10. NHS trusts should:
    put in place hospital-wide systems of care so that patients with suspected or confirmed coronary heart disease receive timely and appropriate investigation and treatment to relieve their symptoms and reduce their risk of subsequent coronary events.

Standard 11: Heart failure

11. Doctors should:
    arrange for people with suspected heart failure to be offered appropriate investigations (e.g. electrocardiography, echocardiography) that will confirm or refute the diagnosis. For those in whom heart failure is confirmed, its cause should be identified – treatments most likely to both relieve their symptoms and reduce their risk of death should be offered.

Standard 12: Cardiac rehabilitation

12. NHS trusts should:
    put in place protocols/systems of care so that, prior to leaving hospital, people admitted to hospital suffering from coronary heart disease have been invited to participate in a multidisciplinary programme of secondary prevention and cardiac rehabilitation. The aim of the programme will be to reduce their risk of subsequent cardiac problems and to promote their return to a full and normal life.

Issues for further consideration

Consider the following protocols and policies for the management of coronary heart disease:

- No smoking policy
- Cycling to work policy
- Safe cycling routes
- Exercise prescription schemes
- Agreed referral criteria for patients with coronary heart disease to be seen by a specialist
- Agreed referral criteria for patients with suspected heart failure
- Agreed protocol between primary and secondary care for the recruitment and management of patients to a cardiac rehabilitation programme and for the palliative and terminal care of end-stage heart failure
- Agreed protocol between primary and secondary care and the ambulance services for the management of suspected myocardial infarction outside the hospital setting
- Agreed protocols for the management of suspected myocardial infarction within secondary care, including door to needle times
- The ambulance service prioritises 999 calls according to agreed criteria

- All ambulances carry defibrillators
- Agreed referral criteria across all disciplines in secondary care for revascularisation of patients with stable angina.

Which are in place in your organisation? Which are agreed with other partners, e.g. local authorities?

The National Institute for Clinical Excellence

In addition to the internal systems and structures set up by individual organisations, there are other statutory bodies that stand outside the NHS but are associated closely with it, and whose functions are to ensure that the process of clinical governance runs smoothly.

The National Institute for Clinical Excellence (NICE) is a special health authority, established on 1 April 1999, which provides national evidence-based clinical guidelines for local adaptation, clinical audit methodologies and information on good practice. It covers the English and Welsh NHS. The Clinical Standards Board carries out a similar function in Scotland and, at the time of writing, Northern Ireland is still consulting about its structures.

NICE has taken over a range of functions previously undertaken by a number of different organisations and groups funded by the Department of Health, including:

- The National Prescribing Centre appraisals and bulletins
- The clinical guidance contained in PRODIGY (a computer-aided decision support system for GPs to assist in their prescribing practice)
- The National Centre for Clinical Audit
- The *Prescriber's Journal*
- The Department of Health funded National Guidelines Programme and Professional Audit Programme
- Effectiveness bulletins

Another key function is the systematic appraisal of medical interventions (current and new drugs and technologies) and their effect on the NHS. NICE operates by working at the local level with NHS organisations (e.g. trusts, health authorities, primary care groups and patient groups) to facilitate the dissemination of the guidance and, nationally, with the Department of Health, Royal Colleges, academic units and other health care industries to ensure that the appropriate information is fed into further clinical reviews or audit methodologies.

NICE carries out 20–30 appraisals annually of the most significant new and existing interventions as identified by the Department of Health. The various industries, including the pharmaceutical industry, are required to produce evidence of clinical and cost effectiveness of their products. If evidence is not available by the time of the launch of the product, or if the proposed product is potentially of value but the evidence is not sufficient, NICE may recommend that the NHS channels its use through well-controlled research studies for further scrutiny. NICE also publishes 18 guidelines annually.

The process that NICE uses in order to produce authoritative guidance is achieved in six stages:[14]

Stage 1: identification of technologies for assessment

Information on all significant new interventions, including all new medicines and new indications for existing drugs and procedures, is gathered through a 'scanning the horizon' process. This provides an early warning on new and current interventions that are likely to have an impact on the NHS. The scanning function is performed by the University of Birmingham in association with the National Prescribing Centre and Drug Information Pharmacists Group. A number of sources are used for scanning, such as published material, patient groups, contact with similar groups in other countries and informal communication with clinicians and researchers.

The selection criteria for interventions requiring further examination include:

- its overall significance to the national health (NHS and non NHS)
- there being a significant challenge for the introduction of the intervention into the NHS – for example, in terms of financial support and impact on services
- the likelihood of resources being misallocated without considered guidance, e.g. treatments for life-threatening or disabling conditions that currently do not have good treatments, or treatments over which there are major ethical concerns.

Stage 2: collection of the evidence

Research is undertaken to assess the clinical and cost effectiveness of the health interventions selected. In addition to clinical outcomes, information will be sought on other areas such as:

- the estimated impact on quality and length of life
- the estimated average health improvement per treatment initiated

- the net NHS costs associated with this health gain
- any associated government-funded personal social services costs and savings
- whether there are significant differences between patient or population sub-groups
- expected total impact on NHS resources (including manpower resources).

All this information is expected to be produced by the sponsoring pharmaceutical company that is introducing the new drug. In the case of a surgical procedure, where this situation is not applicable, the assessment will be carried out by university academic departments.

In addition, relevant patient groupings and other bodies such as the Department of Health, Welsh Office or NHS bodies will be asked to submit views.

Stage 3: appraisal and guidance

NICE is responsible for Stages 3 and 4. Stage 3 involves the careful consideration of the implications for clinical practice of the evidence collated in Stage 2 concerning clinical and cost effectiveness of specific interventions, and the production of guidance for the NHS.

This is under the auspices of the appraisal group, which has a core membership representing professional, academic, NHS and patient groups, with support from a wide range of specialists for expert advice.

The principle output of the appraisal process is whether the intervention is recommended for routine clinical use in the NHS, and the categories which are proposed follow those developed by the South Western Development and Evaluation Committee:

A) Recommended as clinically cost effective for routine use in the NHS for specific indications or patient sub-groups
B) Recommended only for use in the context of clinical trials to help answer specific questions about cost effectiveness/targeting
C) Not recommended for routine use.

Category A could further be qualified as:

 i) recommended for use by all GPs and specialists
 ii) recommended for use in hospitals and for some GPs
iii) recommended for use only by hospital specialists
iv) recommended for use only in specialist tertiary centres.

For those interventions that potentially have value which do not have sufficient evidence to support a recommendation, NICE will advise further research. The intervention will then only be used as part of a programme of clinical research intended to provide such evidence.

Stage 4: dissemination of the guidance

The recommendations, supported by the production of clinical guidance and a brief summary of the evidence, are sent directly to the NHS. In addition, there may be clinical guidelines and audit methodologies to accompany the guidance, covering all aspects of the management of a condition from self-care through primary care to secondary and specialist tertiary services. It is not intended for NICE to make decisions that should be made locally by clinicians for their own patients. The guidance is not there as a substitute for clinical judgement, but to provide a framework.

Information to patients is also produced in consultation with patient bodies and other organisations such as the Centre for Health Information.

Stage 5: implementation at a local level

Once the guidance is disseminated to the NHS, each organisation is expected to implement the recommendations. The mechanism for this is through the local clinical governance structures (see Chapter 2). PCTs are expected to find funding for new treatments within three months of the publication of NICE guidance.

Stage 6: monitoring the impact of the guidance

Feedback on the impact of the guidance and reviewing the advice, particularly in the light of relevant new research findings, is essential to ensure that the recommendations are constantly updated. In particular, there is close liaison with the Medicines Control Agency, which licenses medicines on the basis of safety, quality and efficacy, and the Medical Devices Agency, which assesses the safety and performance of health care products. The monitoring is through the process of clinical audit and performance assessment.

As NICE develops further, it will begin to deal with other interventions such as screening, health promotion and other public health programmes.

Issues for further consideration

● How does the functioning of NICE affect patients' access to drugs and health technologies?

There are some concerns about the functioning of NICE and its impact on new medicines.[15] One concern is that by creating new barriers to the introduction of innovative new therapies, this effectively introduces rationing of health care by delay. Patients demanding drugs that are banned in the UK may generate a black market for popular drugs such as Sildenafil (Viagra). Some of the information requested, in particular the pharmaco-economic data, is unintelligible to health care decision-makers and may serve to confuse rather than inform.

Further information on NICE, its background, roles and functions can be found on the NICE website: www.nice.org.uk

The Commission for Health Improvement

The Commission for Health Improvement (CHI, set up in April 2000) has a role in supporting the development of high quality clinical practice consistently across the NHS. Its function is to provide national leadership on the principles of clinical governance, and to support those organisations that are having difficulty setting up clinical governance arrangements locally when usual channels have failed.

The Commission has a programme of rolling reviews, in which every NHS trust, including primary care trusts, will be visited over a period of 3–4 years. In each review, evidence will be sought that clinical governance arrangements are working and that the national standards produced by NICE are being followed. Subject to regulation, CHI will be able to publish confidential information without consent if it considers that there is serious risk to the health and safety of patients, or if it feels that the risk and urgency of the exercise demands it.

The core functions of the Commission include:

- the provision of national leadership to develop and disseminate clinical governance principles
- the independent scrutiny of local clinical governance arrangements
- undertaking a programme of reviews to monitor the implementation of the National Service Frameworks and the guidance produced by NICE – for example, it will have the authority to take over the national review work already performed by the Clinical Standards Advisory Group
- helping the NHS to identify and tackle serious or persistent problems
- taking the responsibility, over time, for overseeing and assisting with external incident enquiries.

The Commission works closely with other bodies, such as:

1. The Audit Commission, which was established in 1982 to bring together

local authority auditing in England and Wales under the control of a single independent body and to extend that role to the Health Service. The task is enormous, as the Audit Commission needs to demonstrate and promote the effectiveness of the money spent on public health and social services, which is over £90 billion (15% of the nation's gross domestic product). Every year the Commission asks every NHS trust and health authority what areas would benefit from further examination, collates that information and uses this in its study selection.

2. The Heath Service Commissioner, whose statutory role is to investigate complaints about all NHS services which have not been resolved at a local level.

3. The professional regulatory bodies such as the General Medical Council and the Nursing and Midwifery Council, and so on, whose statutory functions are to guide and regulate the relevant health care professionals.

4. The professional organisations such as the Royal Colleges, which represent their members and in some cases set standards for post-graduate education.

5. The Health and Safety Executive, which routinely inspects organisations and checks on aspects of health and safety, including premises, employees and patients.

6. Social services organisations, such as the Social Services Inspectorate.

In addition to the rolling programme, there will be other triggers to obtaining the involvement of CHI, including requests from NHS bodies themselves or from the Secretary of State for Health to carry out specific investigations.

Although CHI has a 'troubleshooting' function, if there is an issue that requires particular attention, it is the responsibility of the local NHS organisations to ensure that the recommended action plans are followed up. If there are problems with the performance of individual clinicians, the Commission will refer these to the appropriate regulatory body (e.g. the General Medical Council, the Nursing and Midwifery Council, etc.) for further action.

The role of CHI is changing; the government announced in 2002 that, subject to primary legislation, a new single Commission is to be set up to inspect both the public and private health care sectors.[16] This organisation, the Commission for Healthcare Audit and Inspection (CHAI), covers the role of CHI, the Audit Commission and the regulatory private health care role of the National Care Standards Commission. A key function of the body is to explain to the public how NHS resources have been deployed and the impact that this is expected to have on improving services, standards and the health of the population.

Principal functions of the Commission for Healthcare Audit and Inspection[16]

- Inspecting all NHS hospitals
- Licensing private health care provision
- Conducting value for money audits
- Validating published performance assessment statistics on the NHS, e.g. waiting list information
- Publishing star rating reports of NHS organisations, including recommending special measures where there are persistent problems
- Publishing reports on the performance of NHS organisations
- Independent scrutiny of patient complaints
- Publishing an annual report on national progress on health care and how resources have been used, and presenting this to Parliament.

Further information on CHI can be found on the CHI website: www.chi.nhs.uk

The National Clinical Assessment Authority (NCAA)

The National Clinical Assessment Authority (NCAA), a Special Health Authority, was established in April 2001 following the recommendations made in the Chief Medical Officer's reports, *Supporting Doctors, Protecting Patients*[17] and *Assuring the Quality of Medical Practice: Implementing Supporting Doctors, Protecting Patients.*[18]

The role of the NCAA is to provide a support service to the NHS when the performance of an individual doctor causes great concern. The doctor's employers, i.e. health authorities, hospital trusts and primary care trusts, can make referrals to the NCAA. The Authority responds to the concerns by providing advice, taking referrals and carrying out targeted assessments where necessary. The Authority currently serves all NHS doctors working in England only, and doctors working for the prison service. As the role of the NCAA develops, dentists will be included in the remit of the Authority. The arrangements for doctors in Wales are under discussion by the Welsh Assembly at the time of writing.

The NCAA, however, does not take over the role of the employer or function as a regulator. It supports the employer by conducting objective assessments on the individual doctor concerned, and provides advice to the referring NHS organisations on courses of action that would be most appropriate. It does not replace the NHS complaints systems (see Chapter 6).

Once a doctor has been referred to the NCAA, the following process or assessment framework takes place.

Table 1.2 Assessment framework for doctor referred to NCAA

Stage one

- Acceptance of a referral by the employer or a self-referral
- Advice and support is provided, including the exploration of possible local resolution

Stage two

- The Formal Assessment, which has two steps:
  - Acceptance of the referral and the designing and setting up of the assessment
  - The assessment process itself

Stage three

- Reporting back to the referring organisation and appropriate action planning. The report from the NCAA to the referring organisation comments on three areas: the health of the doctor concerned, a clinical psychology assessment and performance.

The NCAA works closely with two other bodies – the General Medical Council (GMC) and the Commission for Health Improvement (CHI) – as part of the whole framework for protecting patients and improving the quality of care.

Whilst CHI assesses the development of clinical governance in all NHS organisations, the NCAA assesses the contribution of individual doctors by addressing individual performance issues. The function of the GMC is to investigate doctors in cases of serious misconduct or health concerns, and to address performance issues of individual doctors which may call into question their fitness to practice, and to remain on the medical register.

The NCAA may recommend a referral to either the GMC or the CHI if concerns are raised which are more appropriate to those bodies. Exceptionally, the Authority itself may make a referral directly to these organisations. In a similar vein, these organisations work closely with the NCAA on issues within its remit.

Further information on the NCAA can be found on the NCAA website: www.ncaa.nhs.uk

The National Patient Safety Agency

The National Patient Safety Agency was set up in July 2001 following the publication of the document *Building a Safer NHS for Patients*.[19] Its role principally is to develop a national reporting system for the recording of adverse health care events (see Chapter 6).

The role of the National Patient Safety Agency:[19]

- to set and maintain standards for reporting for the NHS
- to collect, collate, categorise and code adverse event information from the NHS
- to gather other safety-related information from other sources
- to analyse information and maintain records which will be available to the public
- to provide feedback to organisations and individuals on the main issues identified and on key lessons learned from the reporting system
- to produce solutions to reduce risk and prevent harm for future patients
- to set national goals and targets on reducing risk and on harm prevention
- to promote research on patient safety
- to promote a supportive and constructive reporting culture within the NHS
- to collaborate with other bodies.

The national reporting system is mandatory for both individuals and NHS organisations and, although confidential, is open and accessible.

NHS organisations are required to record the following information relating to adverse events and near misses as part of their risk management systems:[19]

- What happened?
- Where did it happen?
- When did it happen?
- How did it happen?
- Why did it happen?
- What action was taken or proposed?
- What impact did the event have?
- What factors minimised, or could have minimised, the impact of the event?

The process of risk management is discussed further in Chapter 6.

Further information on the National Patient Safety Agency (NPSA) can be found on the NPSA website: www.npsa.nhs.uk

The Modernisation Agency

The Modernisation Agency, a part of the Department of Health, was created in April 2001 to help health care staff redesign local health services in accordance with good practice.[9]

Essentially, the Agency provides a problem-solving service to NHS organisations that require help. The service is a supportive one and local NHS organisations are expected to develop, implement and fund initiatives. The service provided by the Modernisation Agency is as follows:

- To help diagnose problems and to suggest possible solutions
  The Agency has an important role in the assessment of the eligibility of organisations to access the NHS Plan performance fund, which encourages the development of good quality services.[9] It has a formal role alongside the strategic health authorities to determine how the performance fund can be used.

- To provide practical tools and skills training
  One example is the clinical governance training programme provided by the National Clinical Governance Support Team.

- To secure patient and carer involvement
  The Agency provides advice on the securing of patient and carer input to service improvements.

- To co-recreate solutions
  This is otherwise known as 'assisted wheel invention'. The rationale here is that an innovation or best practice does not always transfer well from one organisation to another. It needs to go through a process of adaptation or modification in a new organisation.

- To identify good practice
  This is a core element of the Modernisation Agency's work. NHS organisations can access the good practice databases and publications the Agency holds. An example of such a publication is the *NHS Beacons Learning Handbook*. This lists the services that have been particularly innovative in meeting specific health care needs across all sectors. This can be accessed at the Beacon website: www.nhs.uk/beacons

In addition to identifying areas of good practice from within the NHS, the Agency has developed strategic alliances both nationally and internationally with other organisations that have a quality remit including, for example, CHI, NICE, the Royal Colleges, academic institutions and the European Quality Forum.

The work programme of the Modernisation Agency

- Service modernisation
- Identifying and spreading good practice and recognising achievement
- Supporting performance improvement
- Leadership and management development
- Multidisciplinary development
- Targeting specific groups
- Leading service improvement
- Strategic alliances to support modernisation

The Agency has the following teams to carry out its work:

- The National Patient's Access Team
  This team helps NHS organisations meet the NHS Plan maximum waiting time targets of 3 months for outpatients and 6 months for inpatients by looking at improvements in access to services by patients and at patient pathways across primary, secondary and tertiary care. The 'Action On' Programmes (e.g. Action On cataracts, ENT, dermatology and orthopaedics) and various collaboratives (networks of specialty groups across a number of organisations covering areas such as coronary heart disease, orthopaedics and critical care) are examples of the work done by the team.

- The National Clinical Governance Support Team
  This is a multidisciplinary team which helps NHS organisations develop their systems for implementing clinical governance. The support provided by the team includes a programme to equip clinical teams with practical tools and techniques. In the course of its work the team identifies best practice and aids the dissemination of the lessons learned across the NHS.

- The National Primary Care Development Team
  The main function of this team is to support of all aspects of primary care development, such as the primary care collaborative, medicines management programmes and the healthy communities collaborative, which includes social care.

- The Changing Workforce Programme
  The NHS Plan highlighted the need to develop the skills and capabilities of staff which may involve different ways of working. The role of this team is to address the issues raised. The different ways of working can be categorised into four types:
  - Moving a task up or down a traditional uni-disciplinary ladder – e.g. a

consultant physician providing care previously given by doctors in training
- Expanding the breadth of a job – e.g. a rehabilitation practitioner working across traditional professional divides
- Increasing the depth of a job – e.g. the establishment of nurse and therapy consultants
- New jobs – e.g. combining clinical tasks in a different way.

- The Leadership Centre
  This role of this Centre is to bring together different leadership initiatives which provide development programmes for various targeted groups from clinical and managerial backgrounds. It also aims to cover people who are entering the NHS for the first time at university graduate level. The Centre also supports the work of the NHS University which is expected to be fully established by late 2003.

Further details on the Modernisation Agency can be found on its website: www.nhs.uk/modernnhs

The NHS Performance Assessment Framework

The NHS Performance Assessment Framework is the mechanism for NHS organisations to use to help them monitor the delivery of health services against the plans for improvement.[8] It identifies six main areas in which performance can be measured. It has two main purposes: to improve the health of the population and to provide better care and outcomes for people who use the NHS. It also strengthens the link between service agreements (contracts) and the actual clinical work carried out by clinicians. The framework works at a number of levels; for example, by encouraging the exchange of information between different agencies, by providing a structured agenda for meetings between partners across the local health care systems and by focusing efforts of different organisations in specific areas.

The framework aims to use the following indicators of measurement:

- Health improvement
- Fair access
- Effective delivery
- Efficiency
- User/carer experience
- Health outcome of NHS care.

Table 1.3 The NHS Performance Assessment Framework[8]

Areas	Aspects of performance
I. Health improvement	The overall health of populations, reflecting social and environmental factors and individual behaviour as well as care provided by the NHS and other agencies.
II. Fair access	The fairness in the provision of 'services in relation to need on various dimensions: ● geographical ● socio-economic ● demographic (age, ethnicity, sex) ● care groups (e.g. people with learning difficulties)
III. Effective delivery of appropriate health care	The extent to which services are: ● clinically effective (interventions or care packages are evidence-based) ● appropriate to need ● timely ● in line with agreed standards ● provided according to best practice service organisation ● delivered by appropriately trained and educated staff
IV. Efficiency	The extent to which the NHS provides efficient service, including: ● cost per unit of care/outcome ● productivity of capital estate ● labour productivity
V. Patient/carer experience	The patient/carer perceptions on the delivery of services including: ● responsiveness to individual needs and preferences ● the skill, care and continuity of service provision ● patient involvement, good information and choice ● waiting times and accessibility ● the physical environment, the organisation and courtesy of administrative arrangements
VI. Health outcomes of NHS care	NHS success in using its resources to: ● reduce levels of risk factors ● reduce levels of disease, impairment and complications of treatment ● improve quality of life for patients and carers ● reduce premature deaths

The framework provides the basis for assessing NHS services across a range of dimensions, for example:

- A population group – e.g. a geographical area, ethnic group or social class
- A condition or client group – e.g. coronary heart disease, asthma, diabetes, children, older people etc.
- A service organisation – e.g. PCT or NHS trust

The framework continues to be refined and developed in the context of government policy initiatives. At the time of writing the indicator set contains 49 indicators, including 7 clinically-based indicators at trust level. These indicators also encompass indicators linked to the National Service Frameworks, indicators relevant to primary care and indicators based on the outcomes of the national survey of NHS patients.[20] Although the NHS performance indicators were originally designed for Health Authorities, it is probable that PCTs, given their new role as the 'basic unit' of the NHS locally, will be held to account for these data.[21]

Table 1.4 NHS Performance Indicators – Health Authority Level Indicators (2000)[20]	
I. Health improvement	• Deaths from all causes (for people aged 15–64) • Deaths from all causes (for people aged 65–74) • Deaths from cancer • Deaths from all circulatory diseases • Suicide rates • Deaths from accidents • Deaths from injury from accidents
II. Fair access	• Inpatient waiting list • Adult dental registrations • Early detection of cancer • Number of GPs • Practice availability • Elective surgery rates • Surgery rates – coronary heart disease
III. Effective delivery of appropriate health care	• Childhood immunisations • Inappropriately used surgery • Acute care management • Chronic care management • Mental health in primary care

- Cost-effective prescribing
- Returning home following treatment for a stroke
- Returning home following treatment for a fractured hip

IV. Efficiency
- Day case rate
- Length of stay in hospital
- Maternity unit costs
- Mental health unit costs
- Generic prescribing

V. Patient/carer experience
- Patients who wait less than two hours for emergency admission (through Accident and Emergency)
- Cancelled operations
- Delayed discharge
- First outpatient appointments for which patient did not attend
- Outpatients seen within 13 weeks of GP referral
- Percentage of those on a waiting list for 18 months or more
- Patients' satisfaction

VI. Health outcomes of NHS health care
- Conceptions below age 18
- Decayed, missing and filled teeth in 5-year-old children
- Re-admission to hospital following discharge
- Emergency admissions of older people
- Emergency psychiatric re-admission
- Stillbirths and infant mortality
- Breast cancer survival
- Cervical cancer survival
- Lung cancer survival
- Colon cancer survival
- Deaths in hospital following surgery (emergency admissions)
- Deaths in hospital following surgery (non-emergency admissions)
- Deaths in hospital following a heart attack (ages 35–74)
- Deaths in hospital following a fractured hip

Table 1.5 NHS Performance Indicators – Trust Level Indicators (2000)[20]	
Effective delivery of appropriate health care	● Returning home following treatment for a stroke ● Returning home following treatment for a fractured hip
Health outcomes of NHS health care	● 28 day emergency re-admission ● In-hospital premature deaths (30-day perioperative mortality – emergency admission) ● In-hospital premature deaths (30-day perioperative mortality – non-emergency admission) ● In-hospital premature deaths (30-day mortality following acute myocardial infarction) ● Deaths following fractured neck of femur

All of the indicators outlined above are based on statistics that are currently collected, through, for example, the Office for National Statistics, Common Information Core, Cancer Registries, Hospital Episode Statistics, Waiting Times returns, Prescription Pricing Authority PACT data and so on.

For the indicator set to be of most value, the information should enable NHS organisations to benchmark their performance in comparison with each other, so that patients across the country have access to the same high standards of care.

In addition to indicators for personal social services, there are also three 'interface' indicators which support joint performance by the NHS and social services.

NHS performance ratings

The NHS Plan proposed a system of measures to help the public assess the performance of NHS organisations, known as NHS performance ratings.[9] The ratings cover all NHS trusts in England. The government has the responsibility of setting the priorities and key targets and CHI (and subsequently CHAI) is responsible for the development of the methodology and the publication of the ratings. The targets cover key areas such as *NHS Plan* priorities (e.g. waiting times, cancelled operations and hospital cleanliness) and indicators which have a clinical focus, a patient focus and a capacity and capability focus. The reports from the CHI (CHAI) reviews are also taken into account in the star rating assessment. Some of the performance ratings are based on the performance indicators.

Trusts are then rated according to one of four categories (see Table 1.6).[22]

Table 1.6 Rating system of NHS trusts	
Three stars	Trusts with the highest levels of performance
Two stars	Trusts that are performing well overall, but have not quite reached consistently high standards
One star	Trusts which generate cause for concern
Zero stars	Trusts which have shown the poorest levels of performance

It should be noted that where a trust has a low performance rating, it does not necessarily mean that the services are unsafe, or that it does not provide some very good care, often under difficult circumstances.

Further information on the NHS performance ratings can be obtained from: www.doh.gov.uk/performanceratings

Summary

It can be seen that clinical governance sits together with a number of quality initiatives as part of a larger programme for improving health care. The essence of the process is that it is multifaceted and multidisciplinary, with no single professional (nurse, doctor, professional allied to medicine or manager within the NHS) taking the burden or ignoring the responsibility for quality improvement. In the ensuing chapters the key elements of clinical governance will be developed further, not only providing some illustrations but also highlighting some of the issues which may take time to resolve. It should be noted that although some of the examples in the next chapters come from organisations that have changed, the principles remain the same.

References

1. The Secretary of State for Health 1997 The new NHS: modern, dependable. The Stationery Office, London
2. The Secretary of State for Health 1998 A first class service: quality in the new NHS. NHS Executive, London
3. NHS Executive (South Thames) 1997 Review of cervical cancer screening services at Kent and Canterbury Hospitals. NHS Executive, London
4. World Health Organisation 1993 The principles of quality assurance [report on a WHO meeting]. WHO, Geneva
5. Report of the review of patient-identifiable information, chaired by Dame Fiona Caldicott 1997 Department of Health, London
6. The clinical governance support unit: www.cgsupport.org

7. Department of Health 2002 Improvement, expansion and reform: the next 3 years, priorities and planning framework 2003–2006. www.doh.gov.uk/planning 2003-2006/improvementexpansionreform.pdf

8. NHS Executive 1999 The NHS performance assessment framework. NHS Executive, London

9. Department of Health 2000 The NHS plan, a plan for investment, a plan for reform. The Stationery Office, London

10. Department of Health, Welsh Office, Scottish Office Home and Health Department, Northern Ireland Department of Health and Social Services 1998 Report on confidential enquiries into maternal deaths in the United Kingdom, 1994-96. Stationery Office, London

11. Department of Health 1998 Smoking kills: a white paper on tobacco. The Stationery Office, London

12. Department of Health 1998 National service framework: coronary heart disease, emerging findings. The Stationery Office, London

13. Department of Health 2000 National service framework for coronary heart disease: modern standards and service models. Department of Health, London

14. NICE Faster access to modern treatment: how NICE appraisal will work. http://www.nice.org.uk

15. Jones A King's Fund policy paper [unpublished]

16. NHS Executive 2002 Delivering the NHS Plan, next steps on investment, next steps on reform. The Stationery Office, Londoon

17. Department of Health 1999 Supporting doctors, protecting patients: a consultation paper on preventing, recognising and dealing with poor performance of doctors in the NHS in England. The Stationery Office, London

18. Department of Health 2001 Assuring the quality of medical practice: implementing supporting doctors, protecting patients. The Stationery Office, London

19. The NHS Confederation 2001 Building a safer NHS for patients [briefing]. NHS Confederation Publications, London

20. NHS Executive 2000 Improving quality and performance in the new NHS, NHS performance indicators. Health Service Circular 2000/023

21. Department of Health 2001 Shifting the balance of power within the NHS: securing delivery. [www.doh.gov.uk/shiftingthebalance] Department of Health, London

22. Department of Health 2001 NHS performance ratings: acute trusts, specialist trusts, ambulance trusts, mental health trusts 2001/02. Department of Health, London

2

Structure and accountability

Clinical governance as part of corporate governance

Clinical governance is now firmly established as a statutory duty of all NHS organisations and, as such, requires a similar level of responsibility and accountability throughout the hierarchy to that relating to financial matters and other non-clinical areas. Figure 2.1 shows the inter-relationship between clinical governance and other systems of internal control within NHS organisations.

The financial management systems and non-clinical areas together form the Controls Assurance Standards which enable an NHS trust to demonstrate that it is in a position to sign the Statement of Internal Control, showing that an effective internal control framework exists.[1]

In addition to the lines of accountability and responsibility leading up to the Board, there are other areas in common such as risk management and health and safety, infection control, evidence-based care (which includes clinical and cost effectiveness) and many more. It therefore makes sense to link the clinical with the non-clinical areas in terms of ensuring that the outcomes are good and that public money has been well spent.

What is corporate governance?

A number of reports commissioned in the early 1990s by the United Kingdom government (including the Cadbury report on controls assurance[2] and the report of the Nolan committee on public accountability[3]) following failures in government and private sector processes resulted in bringing together a framework for corporate governance for both the private and public sectors. This was formalised in the Code of Conduct and Code of Accountability for NHS organisations.[4]

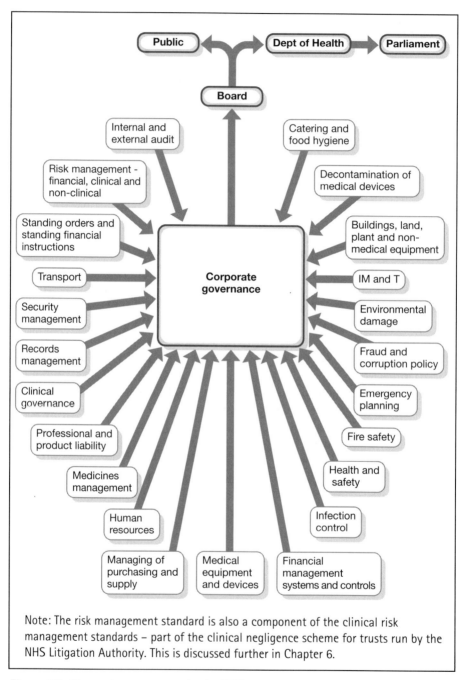

Note: The risk management standard is also a component of the clinical risk management standards – part of the clinical negligence scheme for trusts run by the NHS Litigation Authority. This is discussed further in Chapter 6.

Figure 2.1 Corporate governance in the NHS

The seven principles of the Nolan Report on Standards in Public Life[3] are:

- Selflessness
- Integrity
- Objectivity
- Accountability
- Openness
- Honesty
- Leadership.

NB: The Nolan Standards highlight the qualities required of effective leadership.

The Secretary of State for Health has a statutory responsibility for the health of the population of England, and uses statutory powers to delegate functions to NHS bodies. They are in turn accountable to the Secretary of State for Health and to Parliament. The Chief Executive of the NHS and the NHS Executive are responsible for directing the National Health Service, ensuring national policies are implemented through Strategic Health Authorities, NHS trusts and Primary Care Trusts, and for effective stewardship of NHS resources. A similar accountability structure is in place in Wales with the Welsh Assembly, in Scotland with the Scottish Parliament and in Northern Ireland with the Northern Ireland Office.

The aim of corporate governance is to ensure that public service values are placed at the heart of the NHS. The high standards of conduct expected of those who work in the Health Service are based on the recognition that patients come first (established at the inception of the NHS in 1948) and on the accountability to Parliament (the Welsh Assembly, the Scottish Parliament and the Northern Ireland Office for Wales, Scotland and Northern Ireland respectively) and to taxpayers on the effective use of public funds.

There are three crucial public service values that must run through all the work of the NHS[4]: accountability, probity and openness.

Accountability

Every activity performed by people who work in the Health Service must be robust enough to stand up to close parliamentary scrutiny, the judgement of the general public on propriety (i.e. conforming to the appropriate standard of behaviour), and to professional codes of conduct. This includes achieving value for money from the public funds with which they are entrusted.

The accountability process is as follows:

Strategic health authorities and NHS trusts

NHS boards comprise executive and part-time non-executive directors under a part-time Chair who is appointed by the Secretary of State. Together they share the responsibility for all decisions of the board. The Chief Executive is accountable to the Chair and the non-executives for the operation and implementation of the board's decisions.

Primary care trusts

PCTs have a similar accountability structure to strategic health authorities and NHS trusts. In addition, both the Chair of the professional executive committee of the PCT and the Chief Executive of the PCT are accountable to the Chair of the PCT board.

Probity

It is important that there is honesty in dealing with all the assets of the NHS. People in the NHS must demonstrate absolute integrity and a high ethical standard of personal conduct in their decisions affecting patients, staff and suppliers and also in the use of information acquired in the course of their NHS duties.

The Chair of a strategic health authority or trust and the Director of Finance are directly responsible for the organisation's annual accounts.

Openness

The activities within an NHS organisation should be sufficiently transparent to promote confidence between board members and staff (managers and clinicians), patients and the general public. There is a responsibility for responding to staff, patients and suppliers in an impartial manner.

These public service values apply to all who work in the NHS, regardless of their role and function; in particular, all NHS workers have a responsibility to respond to their colleagues, patients and suppliers impartially, to achieve value for money from the public funds with which they are entrusted and to demonstrate high ethical standards. The process should be transparent, with a willingness to open board meetings to the public and to ensure local community participation in other decision-making processes (e.g. in planning processes and service developments). Board members are required to declare their personal interests on a register which is open to the public. When a conflict of interest occurs, the relevant board member should withdraw and play no part in the discussion or decision.

Issues for consideration

Consider the similarities in the public service values and the clinical professional codes of conduct (see Chapter 10).

● Which areas are similar, and which are different?

The statutory framework

The statutory framework provides a mechanism for the business conduct of an NHS organisation. They are formalised in the standing financial instructions and standing orders.

These agreements fulfill the dual role of protecting the NHS organisation's interests and protecting staff from accusations that they have acted less than properly.

The standing orders and standing financial instructions set out formally how the NHS organisation works.

Standing orders include:

● The way business is conducted – for example, board membership and voting rights
● Delegated powers – for example, delegating specific functions of the PCT to a committee or sub-committee, or to an officer of a PCT, which can then be undertaken without further reference to the PCT board
● Declarations of interest – board members must declare interests such as directorships, company ownership, and involvement in any organisations, voluntary or otherwise, which operate in the field of health and social care, to avoid conflicts' of interest
● Tendering and contracting for services – this section governs the stages involved in the proper letting of tenders for purchase of goods and services and building schemes.

Standing financial instructions include:

● Financial management – audit
● Negotiating contracts
● Non-pay expenditure
● Information technology and data protection
● Payments to independent contractors

Issues for consideration

Standing orders state that a conflict of interest must be declared by board members.

● How does this relate to general practitioners who work with the pharmaceutical industry (e.g. have the benefit of a specialist nurse in their practice or carry out research on behalf of a drug company)?

Controls assurance

The Cadbury Report, produced in 1992,[2] recommended that the board of directors of each listed company registered in the United Kingdom should report on the effectiveness of the company's system of internal control. This recommendation applies to the public as well as the private sector. With respect to the NHS this means that the concept of 'controls assurance' requires that every strategic health authority and trust board must be satisfied that systems are in place within the organisation to ensure that risks are properly assessed and managed. A statement accompanying the annual report and accounts should be produced, and acts as confirmation to the general public that the board of directors believes these systems are in place and operating effectively.

The areas covered by the Controls Assurance Statement are shown in Figure 2.1, above.

Accountability for clinical governance

The Chief Executive of a strategic health authority or trust is now obliged to sign two assurance statements on behalf of the board; one for controls assurance and the other for clinical governance to demonstrate probity, accountability and quality across the organisation.

The White Paper *A First Class Service* has indicated that the principles of clinical governance are to 'apply to all those who provide or manage patient care services in the NHS'. Therefore the responsibility is upon clinicians and managers alike to deliver high quality health care.

Both sets of statements are subject to external audit; one for finance (which has been in place since 1991, under section 10 of the NHS and Community Care Act 1990) and the other for the quality of clinical care. For proper financial stewardship, trusts are legally obliged to *ensure* revenue meets outgoing spend (i.e. achieving a balance at the end of the financial year) and to *achieve* the Secretary of State's financial objectives. A similar process needs to be in place for quality of care – i.e. to *achieve quality*. However, it is not entirely clear how quality will be defined for this purpose. There may need to be a level of discretion built into that duty to ensure that individual trusts and PCTs will be open to a major challenge from judicial review when they are balancing the need to impose a duty without exposure to the hazard of extra litigation.

Issues for consideration

- Is it appropriate for a non-specialist, i.e. a non-clinical Chief Executive, to be responsible for the clinical care of an organisation?

There have been some concerns that managers should be held responsible for failures in clinical performance even though they do not have the expert knowledge or the powers to influence clinical practice. However, it has been argued that Chief Executives have for some time (since the last set of NHS reforms in 1991), had the responsibility for the financial performance of their institutions and some may not have had a background in accountancy. Taking the argument further, if the examples of other industries are examined, Chief Executives of large organisations are held responsible, as far as the shareholders are concerned, for the overall performance of their companies, including the performance of the technical aspects (such as engineering or piloting an aeroplane and so on), of which they may have little knowledge. In these situations they are reliant on the technical experts within the company for advice, quality and delivery of the appropriate work. Chief Executives are dependent on the experts within the organisation to deliver on the quality of the product, and yet they are accountable if the standards are not maintained and the return to shareholders is not achieved.

Comments from Chief Executives of NHS organisations concerning their legal responsibilities for clinical performance[5]

- 'Chief Executives are responsible for everything that goes on in a trust anyway. Nothing has changed.'
- 'I have always held myself accountable for all the trust's activities. I have never assumed these things are not my responsibility. What clinical governance might give me is a bit more legitimacy.'
- 'I am confident we will make progress but feel challenged about being able to demonstrate this.'
- 'I don't think I am legally responsible for clinical governance – I don't think I can be sued. I am accountable as a public servant, but I don't think I can be sued for anything that goes wrong in the operating theatre.'
- 'I have never doubted that I was legally responsible for clinical performance since I became Chief Executive. The idea that somehow you can stand aside if there is a clinical disaster is amazing.'
- 'Most Chief Executives I know are naturally very nervous about this [framing of the legislation of the Chief Executive's legal responsibility], and with emergency services under such pressure I do not see any acute Chief Executive being happy or confident about putting their neck on the line.'

Clearly there is a range of responses to the legal responsibility of clinical governance imposed on Chief Executives. The comments reflect the anxiety over the lack of influence managers feel they have over clinical performance. In the past this has often resulted in the dismissal of managers, and this action has not necessarily led to any improvements in clinical practice. How the situation will turn out in the future will depend on how clinical governance evolves.

There is a different set of concerns relating to clinical and corporate governance and possible conflicts for general practitioners as clinicians and members of PCTs. The principles also apply to the other independent contractors (dentists, high street pharmacists and optometrists), albeit to a lesser degree.

Christopher Newdick, Lecturer in Law at the University of Reading (personal communication, 1999) argues that a distinction needs to be made between clinical and corporate governance. He states that the former is concerned with monitoring and regulating the relationship between doctor and patient, by promoting best clinical practice, and the latter supervises the NHS organisations, by ensuring that effective use is made of limited resources and that the conduct of the institution is open and accountable. There is a potential conflict when measures designed to improve the effective use of resources may inhibit clinical discretion. For example, the *Terms of Service for Doctors in General Practice*[6] states, amongst other things, that a doctor shall render to his patients:

- All necessary and appropriate personal medical services of the type usually provided by General Medical Practitioners. This includes the requirement to prescribe any drugs and appliances that in their clinical judgement are needed by a patient
- Referral, where appropriate, to other NHS services and social services.

However, access to services and the prescription of new and expensive drugs are dependent on the amount of funding available. PCTs are obliged to remain within their unified budgets and any overspends in the indicative prescribing budgets are to be managed within the overall resource envelope.

There is, of course, the option of borrowing from the following year's budget; however, this does not tackle the underlying problem of overspending. Until the *Terms of Service for Doctors in General Practice* is reviewed in the light of this potential conflict, the way is open for difficulties ahead.

Leadership by the board

The board of an NHS organisation has a very important role in leading cultural change and ensuring top-down support for frontline staff in the implementation of clinical governance processes. Various CHI clinical governance reviews have highlighted the leadership roles of non-executive directors in trusts.[7]

Examples of leadership roles of non-executive directors in trusts[7]

- Reviewing and restructuring the way clinical governance is managed within an organisation
- Demonstrating a depth of understanding about clinical governance issues and leading key areas of sensitivity (e.g. consent for organ donation)
- Supporting improvements to increase patient involvement and consultation
- Chairing clinical governance committees.

It is important that the board of an NHS organisation takes 'time out' to consider its role in supporting clinical governance. Poorly led organisations which have inadequate systems in place cannot support the delivery of effective care.

The NHS Clinical Governance Support Team has identified the key characteristics of successful board teams.[7]

- The most important challenge is to get the right people into the right positions
- Do not focus primarily on what to do to become great; focus equally on what not to do and what to stop doing
- Boards must maintain unwavering faith that they can and will prevail, and at the same time have the discipline to confront the most brutal facts of their current reality.

Leaders within an organisation

Successful implementation of clinical governance within an NHS organisation depends upon leaders who are able to inspire and motivate others. Leaders occur throughout an organisation and are not necessarily the people at the top of the hierarchy, or just managers. According to Bennis 'Leaders are people who do the right thing, managers are people who do things right... Leadership is the cap to transforming vision into reality'.[8]

Styles of leadership

Four styles of leadership have been identified in the literature:[9]

- transactional (task accomplishment)

- transformational (concerned with interpersonal relations)
- renaissance (empowerment and influencing health care policy)
- connective (a bridge between the transformational and renaissance styles).

Transactional leadership has been the traditional style that has been used by the NHS in the past and this was viewed as important in order to maintain stability and to achieve the goals of the organisation. Transformational leadership, however, is the style that is suited to the current environment of change as it embraces and encourages innovation and change, qualities that are essential in developing and implementing clinical governance. It could be argued that renaissance and connective leadership styles are aspects of transformational leadership that have been developed further; for example, influencing health care policy is an increasingly important role that leaders within the NHS can play.

Clinical governance reports

An essential mechanism for monitoring the impact of clinical governance in an organisation is to have regular reports to the board indicating the areas of progress and remedial action in the areas where improvement is necessary.

An indication of what should be reported as a minimum is the expected scope of the annual reports required for 1999/2000 for all NHS organisations. It is anticipated that the reports will develop in sophistication and complexity as clinical governance evolves. The minimum requirements are:[10]

- An explanation of the leadership, accountability and working arrangements for implementing clinical governance
- Work to ensure that clinical decision making is increasingly evidence based, on a local level and nationally, with the recommendations of the National Service Frameworks and NICE guidelines
- Progress on integrated planning for quality, including information establishing explicit links to Health Improvement and Modernisation Programmes (HIMPs) (now called Local Development Programmes) and National Service Frameworks, if appropriate
- Progress on continuing professional development and life-long learning, and designing ways in which staff development, educational and workforce solutions are being used to support clinical governance
- Participation in, and impact of, multidisciplinary audit programmes – including national specialty and sub-specialty audits – and national confidential enquiries
- The identification of particular services in which there are specific

shortfalls in quality and of deficits in other clinical governance support mechanisms (e.g. risk management, clinical audit etc.)
- Evidence of active working with the public, users of services and their carers
- An account of the mechanisms that have been established to ensure that lessons are being learned from complaints, adverse incidents and enquiries into services.

Models of clinical governance

The principles of clinical governance outlined in *A First Class Service* state that there must be clear lines of responsibility and accountability for the overall quality of clinical care within an NHS organisation. These should include the appointment of a designated senior clinician, ideally at board level, to ensure that systems and structures are in place to enable the board to discharge their responsibilities.

Clinical governance committees have been set up using a number of different approaches. The starting point has been the assessment of the various groups and committees currently in place within the organisation, which have then been modified to meet the new criteria (see also Chapter 3).

Joint clinical/corporate governance committees

In some trusts a single governance committee has been created as a sub-committee of the board and this has the joint remit of clinical and corporate governance.[11] This type of committee has replaced an existing audit committee, which looks at financial accountability and probity of the organisation, and has extended the remit to include clinical governance.

In accordance with sub-committees of boards, a non-executive director takes the chair. This provides them with an opportunity to get involved in the kinds of issues they came into the NHS to influence, but in which they do not necessarily have the knowledge or expertise required. A major risk is that non-executive directors may be in danger of becoming peripheral to the process, and so weaken the accountability process.

Who is the board lead for clinical governance?

This responsibility has tended to fall on the shoulders of the Medical Director (consultant or general practitioner as appropriate) for a trust board and PCT, and the Director of Public Health for a strategic health authority. If the Director of Nursing is involved, it is usually as a joint role with a medical colleague. Although it is appropriate for the lead to be clinically qualified, the small representation from nurses raises the issue of the involvement of other clinical professionals and the expectations of working in a multidisciplinary way.

A key theme of the reforms is multidisciplinary and collaborative working. Implementation of clinical governance offers an opportunity to do this by ensuring that the various professional groups are able to provide feedback on their work to the main clinical governance committee.

The shape of the clinical governance committee and supporting structures

The clinical governance committee or its equivalent should ensure the involvement of the relevant groupings or functions which contribute to this area in order to build up the overall picture. As discussed above, some clinical governance committees are combined with corporate governance committees in an attempt to ensure a smooth line of accountability to the board. Other trusts have chosen alternative paths and have different members, ranging from clinical directors and relevant managers to including representatives from other organisations such as the local PCT and other NHS trusts. In a similar vein, some PCTs are requesting input from their local trusts, as well as from social services and user and carer representatives.

In its discussion document,[12] North Thames Regional Office proposed five essential building blocks to clinical governance which included clinical audit, clinical effectiveness, risk management, quality assurance and the development of staff and organisations. To nurture such an environment, the paper continued, NHS organisations needed to:

- encourage team work and collaborative standard setting
- empower all clinicians
- develop shared information to monitor standards
- use an appropriate mix of incentives and sanctions.

A few years down the track, the above criteria still hold true.

Within NHS trusts, the approach to the support for clinical governance is based on the structures already in place for quality – for example: performance indicators; clinical risk management; complaints; waiting list projects; clinical audit; patient information initiatives and quality programmes (which include pressure ulcers, infection control, nutrition, falls in older people, etc.), health and safety and so on. Many of the groups have differing terms of reference and accountabilities.

The links between education and training, such as postgraduate medical

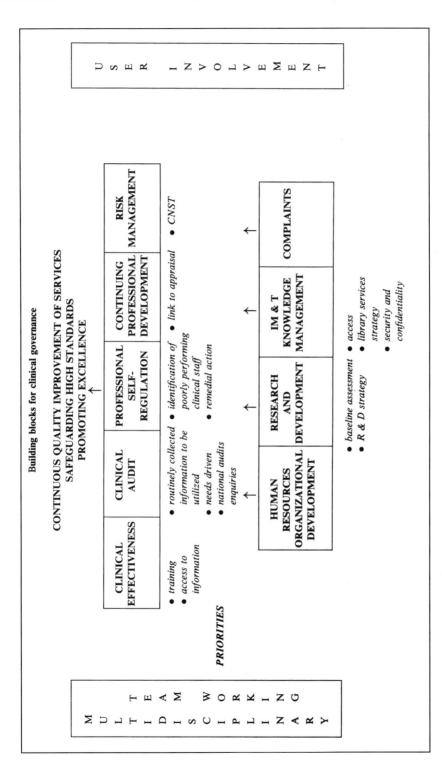

Table 2.1 Clinical governance structure from South Warwickshire Combined Healthcare NHS Trust

centres for doctors and training and development for nurses and allied health professionals etc., are being strengthened with clinical governance structures. In addition, greater support on research initiatives and access to information on evidence-based practice is being provided.

For mental health and learning disabilities trusts, the challenge is to engage with social services colleagues, as there is a great overlap in the provision of care in some cases. This may require a change of the 'clinical governance' title to something that has less of a medical meaning.

However the supporting structures are brought together for the purposes of clinical governance, the essential step is to align them to the clinical directorate structure for implementation.

The picture is not so straightforward for primary care. Although PCTs tend to be regarded as a single, coherent organisation, in reality they are made up of independent medical contractors whose practices have employed staff, who are, in turn, working with community services colleagues under the same PCT banner. For clinical governance to work in this setting, differing needs should be recognised and met. Each PCT has an appointed lead for clinical governance on the board; however, these clinicians need to work closely with the clinical governance leads for the individual practices.

A model for the development of clinical governance in primary care has been proposed by Baker and colleagues (1999).[13] It describes the activities that could be undertaken as part of clinical governance to cover the tasks of defining, accounting for and improving quality at three levels – the health professional, the primary health care team and the PCG/T. Each grouping would need to define and agree aspects of quality that are relevant to particular professional activities.

A key element of the model is ensuring that the system of accountability is transparent and at the same time that careful consideration of the rules for confidentiality of information (including the point at which this is broken to protect patients) is made. That individual health professionals are accountable for their own performance is clear; however, primary health care teams and the PCG/T are also accountable both for performance and its improvement to the strategic health authority and the local community.

Issues for consideration

Consider the structure for clinical governance set up in your organisation.

- Are the key people involved?
- Does the clinical governance lead inspire your support?
- Do you know what you are supposed to do?

Table 2.2 A model of clinical governance (adapted from Baker et al, reprinted with permission from the BMJ Publishing Group)[13]

The figures 1-4 denote the levels of development of primary care groups (1-2) and primary care trusts (3-4)

Individual health care professionals

Quality	1. GMC/NMC standards, GP terms and conditions of service 2. Individual competency skills in consultations 3. Professional development 4. Patient views, evidence-based practice
Accountability	1. Reports on training undertaken, complaints, participation in clinical audit. Persistent poor performance dealt with 2. Audit of competencies and skills 3. Relevant anonymised audit reports to patients 4. Patients involved in choosing audit topics/assessing performance
Quality improvement	1. Improvement in consultation performance 2. Clinical audit results 3. Personal appraisal 4. Personal development plans

Primary health care team

Quality	1. NICE recommended topics 2. Local priorities e.g. HIMP 3. Health needs assessment 4. Patient involvement, evidence-based practice
Accountability	1. Report on assessment and audit of NICE topics 2. Participation in audits 3. Publication of clinical audit results within NHS 4. Relevant anonymised results of audits available to patients
Quality improvement	1. Multidisciplinary protocols in use 2. Multidisciplinary audit taking place 3. Practice professional development plan 4. Fully implemented quality improvement programme including systems to identify obstacles to change, e.g. through the use of integrated care pathways

Primary care group/Primary care trust	
Quality	1. One or two topics from NICE, National Service Framework or HImP
	2. More NICE, National Service Framework or HImP topics
	3. Comprehensive population health needs assessment with clear objectives
	4. Patient involvement, systematic evidence-based practice
Accountability	1. Performance data reported to strategic health authority Persistently poor performing teams and individuals are supported to improve
	2. Annual report on quality of care issued to local health and social services and to Commission for Health Improvement
	3. Annual quality report available to the public. Participation in accreditation schemes for groups
	4. Patient involvement in assessing the quality of service
Quality improvement	1. Findings of audits on topics fed back to practice teams and plans for improvement made
	2. Audit findings compared with those of other groups, obstacles to improvement identified
	3. Wide range of methods used to overcome obstacles for change
	4. Comprehensive quality management system in place throughout the group

Clinical governance leads have a challenging task ahead of them to ensure the establishment of a new culture within their organisations to allow clinical governance to flourish. The culture (shared beliefs, values and commitment) should be such that good quality is prized and a sense of accountability is instilled in clinicians and managers for achieving high standards. A major aspect is the commitment of all involved to:[14]

- meeting the needs of individual patients
- improving the health of the public
- clinical quality
- clinical accountability
- multidisciplinary learning and development
- open and reflective practice
- respect and support colleagues
- an inclusive approach to working in partnership.

Clinical governance leads need to contribute by:

- demonstrating commitment from the top
- developing corporate responsibility for quality
- shaping and communicating enthusiastically the local vision for clinical governance
- facilitating the development of a 'bottom up' approach
- securing an inclusive involvement
- co-ordinating and staying in touch with local arrangements
- ensuring that robust systems are in place or are being developed.

Setting up committees to implement clinical governance in organisations is relatively straightforward. Setting up systems to improve quality and to show accountability is another, more complex, process. The next chapter discusses the importance of empowering clinicians and the engagement of key players to ensure the successful implementation of clinical governance.

References

1. Controls Assurance Standards 2001-2002 http://tap.ukwebhost.eds.com/doh/rm5.nsf/AdminDocs/CAStandards?OpenDocument
2. 'Cadbury report': Report of the committee on the financial aspects of corporate governance 1992. Gee, London
3. Report on standards in public life, chaired by Lord Nolan 1995. HMSO, London
4. Department of Health 1994 Corporate governance in the NHS: code of conduct, code of accountability. Department of Health, London
5. Millar B 1999 Carry that weight. Health Service Journal 18 February: 22-27
6. Department of Health 1989 Terms of service for doctors in general practice. Department of Health, London
7. Wall D, Halligan A, Deighan M et al 2002 Leadership, strategy and clinical governance, nexus backgound. NHS Modernisation Agency 4
8. Bennis W 1990 Why leaders can't lead. Jossey-Bass, San Francisco
9. Ewens A 2002 The nature and purpose of leadership. In: Howkins E, Thornton C (eds) Managing and leading innovation in healthcare. Baillière Tindall, London
10. NHS Executive 1999 Clinical governance: quality in the new NHS. Health Service Circular 1999/065
11. Walshe K 1999 Clinical governance and NHS boards: the emerging picture. HMSC School of Public Policy, University of Birmingham Newsletter 5(2)
12. The Department of Public Health, NHS Executive, North Thames Regional Office 1998 Clinical governance in North Thames. NHSE North Thames, London
13. Baker R, Lakhani M, Fraser R et al 1999 A model for clinical governance in primary care groups. British Medical Journal 318: 779-783
14. Rotherham G, Martin D 1999 Clinical governance in primary care: policy into practice, findings. The NHS Confederation, London

3

Achieving change in clinical governance

The key to the successful implementation of clinical governance and the setting up of appropriate systems within an NHS organisation is the way in which the different quality initiatives are brought together under one cohesive structure or banner. The smooth co-ordination of the individual components identified in the White Paper *A First Class Service*,[1] must be seen to be working more effectively than the sum of the parts. An important step in this process is how the change in culture, systems and people's behaviour can be brought about.

Setting up systems for clinical governance

There is a temptation, as with any new project, to move speedily to set up new structures, working groups, committees and so on, and to assign new roles and responsibilities without a careful examination of what currently exists (for example, current skills and expertise) or having a proper understanding of some of the relationships and cultural issues that may act as barriers to implementation.

As mentioned before, clinical governance is not a new concept. It is a framework upon which to hang different quality initiatives. Many of the systems required for clinical governance already exist within organisations, and these should be used as the building blocks upon which to begin the process. Close examination of the working of some organisations may actually reveal an effective structure for clinical governance, possibly known under a different name. Others may need to develop or strengthen certain activities.

Issues for consideration

Consider which quality initiatives are already in place in your organisation.

- Which require strengthening?
- What are the barriers that need addressing?

Before management structures are set up, it is sensible to carry out an audit of systems and structures currently in place. Ascertaining the position, even once the systems have been set up, is an essential part of the process, the aim being to improve quality continuously supported by regular review.

The checklist below is an example of an approach to such an audit (adapted from *Guidance for Nurses on Clinical Governance* [2]). This could be used at any level of the organisation, whether at clinical directorate, primary care trust board or local clinical team level.

Table 3.1 A quality audit (from Guidance for Nurses on Clinical Governance [2])				
Elements	Are the right frameworks in place?	Are they working well?	How could they be improved?	Points for action
Multi-professional clinical audit				
Evidence-based practice				
Clinical supervision				
Management and systematic learning from complaints				
Clinical risk management				
Clinical incident reporting				
Management of adverse events				
Continuing professional development				
Clinical leadership development				

Elements	Are the right frameworks in place?	Are they working well?	How could they be improved?	Points for action
Patient/user feedback systems				
Identification and management of poor clinical performance				
Quality of data for monitoring clinical care				

TABLE 3.2 Processes for clinical governance[2]

Processes	Are the frameworks in the right place?	Are they working well?	How could they be improved?	Points for action
Patient/user focused approach				
Integrated approach to managing and improving quality				
Effective multidisciplinary team work				
Information sharing and networking				
Open and supportive culture; learning from mistakes				

The next step is to examine the processes necessary for clinical governance to flourish; that is, to identify and understand the culture within which clinicians are working. Here, the importance of multidisciplinary working relationships, networking, collaboration and practical support at all levels will make or break the system by either setting up barriers or facilitating the process of quality improvement. The commitment of the board and all clinicians and other non-clinical staff in the organisation in providing an enabling environment is essential. The concept of shared governance is helpful here. In this situation, members of important committees, particularly those with decision-making powers, should be elected as true representatives of their occupational groups rather than delegates by the top management team. The processes to consider are illustrated in Table 3.2.[2]

The third step is to identify the infrastructure needed to support clinical governance. This is about allowing clinicians the opportunity to participate actively in the process and to identify the individual training and development needs of all staff.

Infrastructure	Are the frameworks in the right place?	Are they working well?	How could they be improved?	Points for action
Time allowed for staff to get involved				
Access to continuing professional development				
Access to information – libraries, journals, guidelines etc.				

Table 3.3 Infrastructure to support clinical governance[2]

On a larger organisational level, the audit should address the following issues:[3]

- An analysis of the organisation's strengths and weaknesses in relation to current performance. This should be an honest assessment undertaken by the key people involved.
- Any problematic services using, if possible, objective data or information from users of services and from the agencies that make the referrals.
- An assessment of the extent to which appropriate information systems for collecting data are in place.

- Checking for deficiencies in key processes (e.g. risk management, complaints, multidisciplinary clinical audit, involvement of patients).
- Ensuring that there is a connection between quality activities – e.g. clinical audit, complaints and clinical risk management.
- Establishing links with national and local priorities identified in the Health Improvement and Modernisation Programmes and National Service Frameworks.
- Allow time for staff to understand and own the process.

Once the audit of current key processes and infrastructure has been undertaken, it is appropriate to examine the response of people within an organisation or team to the implementation of clinical governance.

Engaging stakeholders in setting up clinical governance systems

As with any proposed change, at any level and in any situation, most people's reaction is to resist that change. This resistance is exacerbated further if that change is compulsory. This is the situation with clinical governance; it is a statutory responsibility that individuals and organisations must implement. In reality, it is a complex process that requires the winning of many hearts and minds, and there are many ways in which the changes can be introduced into a team or organisation that will have varying degrees of success.

Motivation

A key factor is an individual's motivation to change, particularly in the work setting. It is usually straightforward to think up arguments for actions that will benefit oneself, such as access to training or working in a particular way, but the reactions of colleagues may not be quite so easy to identify.

The challenge facing the lead for clinical governance in any organisation cannot be under-estimated. Encouraging others to look at and take up new and different ways of delivering clinical care can be an enormous task. Motivation is a very difficult thing to measure in practice, although it is recognisable in ourselves and others at work and at home. Motivation is a vast and complex topic, and it is only possible to discuss a few key ideas in this chapter.

There are essentially two ways of looking at motivation; one is based on the individual's basic needs and the other is based on the forces that affect motivation.

The needs theories

In 1954 an American psychologist, Abraham Maslow,[4] developed a system for looking at motivation. He postulated that motivation was dependent on the desire to satisfy various levels of needs, and that people conduct themselves in a way that fulfils their needs. Once a need has been satisfied, it ceases to motivate the individual. So, for example, if an individual's job does not satisfy his or her cognitive needs (the desire to know, understand and explore) then the motivation to look at ways of improving the quality of clinical practice through audit is not there. Maslow's hierarchy of needs is shown diagrammatically in Figure 3.1.

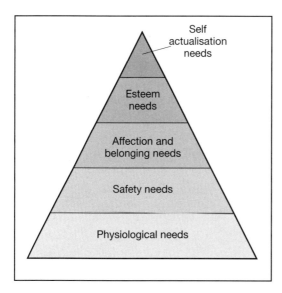

Figure 3.1 Maslow's hierarchy of needs

In terms of motivation at work, Maslow's hierarchy of needs can be interpreted in the following way (adapted from How to motivate people by T. Dell and *She Who Dares Wins* by E. Gillibrand and J. Mosley:[5]

- Physiological needs. The basic human need is survival. The core of employee satisfaction is to:
  - work for an efficient manager
  - think for oneself.
- Emotional safety. The next level of need is security. At this level employees need to:
  - see the end result of their work
  - be involved in interesting work.

Demotivation could arise from job insecurity or backbiting/bullying from colleagues.

- Affection and belonging. The third level of need is belonging. For belonging, employees need to:
  - be listened to
  - be informed.

Demotivation could arise from an unwelcoming workplace or isolation at work.

- Self-esteem. The fourth level is prestige. For prestige, employees need:
  - respect
  - recognition
  - positive feedback
  - opportunity to use untapped skills.
- Self-actualisation. The final level is self-fulfillment. At this level, employees need:
  - a challenge
  - the opportunity to experiment with ideas
  - skill development.

Issues for consideration

- Using the hierarchy of needs model, at each level, consider possible examples of a need that motivates you.
- How helpful is the diagram in explaining your behaviour at work?

Although the examples of the types of needs in Maslow's model can be identified by most people, they are not always given the same relative importance. In practice there is a movement up and down the hierarchy, depending on the different stages of life and career at which individuals find themselves.

Another way of looking at motivation is a theory constructed by Herzberg and colleagues.[6] Here, the suggestion is that in any work situation there are factors that satisfy and those that dissatisfy.

Motivating factors – can lead to satisfaction (i.e. Why work harder?)	Hygiene factors – can lead to dissatisfaction, if lacking (i.e. Why work here?)
Achievement	Salary
Recognition	Being under supervision
Work itself	Work relationships
Responsibility	Company policy
Advancement	Working conditions
New tasks/responsibilities	Job security

Interestingly enough, Herzberg found that pay itself was not a prime satisfier, but can be a dissatisfier if lacking. The key argument is that motivation is essentially a subjective phenomenon – i.e. how the individual concerned perceives it is what matters.

Issues for consideration

- Consider your own work situation. List the factors that satisfy and those that cause dissatisfaction – don't forget the added factors required of you under clinical governance. Give each factor a ranking from 1 to 3, with 3 being the greatest strength.
- What is it that motivates you the most?
- What demotivates you?

The motivation of individuals cannot work in isolation and without interaction of others. McClelland and his colleagues[7] looked at the way people think in many cultures and in many sections of society. Responses were classified into three areas representing an identifiable human motive or need. They are:

- the need for affiliation
- the need for power
- the need for achievement.

People are motivated by various combinations of these needs.

The need for affiliation

The person who demonstrates a high need for affiliation will tend to be more concerned with developing and maintaining relationships than with making decisions. This type of individual is often seen as an ineffective helper, probably because they do not concentrate on the task in hand. In other words they are usually concerned about how they will be perceived by others, and try too hard to please instead of attending to a piece of work which requires a concentrated approach. This characteristic is probably present in most people, and is an important component in team working, but is rarely dominant in successful, ambitious individuals.

The need for power

A high need for power will by itself lead to a situation rather like a military dictatorship. Here, many demands are made by the individual, with little or no involvement of other members of the team in the process of making decisions and implementation. Combining this need with, for example, the need for achievement, can lead to productive and satisfying results. This characteristic tends to be found in some degree or other in managers and doctors.

The need for achievement

The type of individual who exhibits this characteristic tends to like personal responsibility, takes moderate and calculated risks and requests feedback on how they are doing. There is a strong correlation between a high need for achievement and high levels of performance. However, if not moderated by the other needs, people with a high need for achievement may become too individualistic to be very successful in any organisation where other points of view need to be expressed.

These are major categories of needs, and the list could go on. Individual needs vary widely from one person to another. In addition, the relative importance of each need can change over time, depending on external circumstances.

Issues for consideration

- Consider three of your colleagues who work in the same team as yourself. Score against them the three needs identifies by McClellend (power, affiliation and achievement). Indicate the strength of these characteristics using + to indicate a low need and +++ for a high need in their day-to-day work. Check these perceptions with your colleagues.
- Repeat this exercise for three colleagues at the top of the organisation (e.g. Chief Executive, Medical Director etc.). How are the two sets of assessments different?

The process or cognitive theories

Process or cognitive theories consider the important relationship between outcome and effort or performance. Vroom[8] developed the expectancy theory in which, for change to occur, the person concerned must believe that the effort will increase the possibility of obtaining the reward.

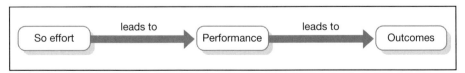

Figure 3.2 The process of cognitive theories

In the NHS, outcomes are rewarded, not the effort or performance; these outcomes can be positive or negative and may not necessarily be financial in nature.

In their goal theory, Latham and Locke[5] state that motivation and performance are greater when:

- individuals are set specific goals
- the goals are difficult but accepted
- there is feedback on performance.

The NHS has been set goals through the statutory duty of clinical governance, but these have not been arrived at through a consensus. These goals have been imposed from above, although a 'bottom up' approach is expected, for which there is some in-built flexibility – e.g. there is a choice of national and local priority subjects that NHS organisations can use.

Going through the various exercises clearly demonstrates that what motivates human beings is not satisfied by any one particular theory. Motivation is derived from a complex interaction of a number of factors and what is a motivating factor for one person may not be so for another.

It is important to note that leadership style has an impact on the performance of individuals within an organisation (this is discussed further in Chapter 9).

The pressures for change

Machiavelli said: 'There is nothing more difficult to carry out, nor more doubtful of success, nor more dangerous to handle, than to initiate a new order of things.' This statement is applicable to major policy initiatives ranging from risk management systems covering a whole hospital to new clinical guidelines for a medical team to changing the format of GP referral letters. It is certainly true of clinical governance. The wide-ranging expectations of clinical governance make the process of change a high-risk business, and there is a danger of leaving many people behind.

There are three types of change: routine, improvement and innovation.[9] Clinical governance falls into the improvement and innovation categories of change.

Meadows and colleagues[10] identified three main components that are necessary to bring about change in an organisation of any size.

A dissatisfaction with the current situation

The feeling of dissatisfaction needs to be shared by a reasonable proportion of the organisation or team. This is difficult to engender with a large scale change that is obligatory. However, it is only when people themselves realise the probable consequences of letting the current situation drift out of their control that they will be stimulated into thinking about more desirable alternatives. In the area of clinical governance, the probable driver will be the possibility of being left behind and having systems imposed upon individuals and teams without consultation.

An agreed vision of a more desirable future

If everyone in a team or organisation has a different view of what is required, then change will not come about. A number of key opinion leaders need to share (i.e. agree upon) a common vision. Creating this common vision is a challenging task for anyone, and requires an understanding of the political processes and relationships within the team or organisation. This has, to a certain extent, already been mapped out by the government's policy on clinical governance; however the detail and the change management process still needs to be done on a local organisational level.

Working out the first steps

Practical steps need to be taken to turn the vision into reality. This requires a clear, well thought out action plan, which has been communicated effectively to the team or throughout an organisation. This best achieved by taking some time out and working with an independent facilitator. Without the action plan it will be immensely difficult to achieve the different way of working envisaged. This is the role of the clinical governance lead and the clinical governance committee: to provide clarity and direction for the whole organisation.

When these three ingredients are present, the costs of change need to be identified. These should clearly include financial and time costs (people learning new clinical skills, or performing audit, are not actually seeing and treating patients), as well as the less tangible elements such as irritation, frustration and the possibility of failure (the new way of working does not seem to be improving the clinical care of patients). Essentially, change is most likely to go ahead if the potential benefits outweigh the costs. The main message therefore, for those who have a responsibility to implement clinical governance, is to think through carefully the arguments for and against the proposed changes. The benefits have been identified already (see Table 3.4); however the major concern is the potential cost in setting up the whole process, although there is scope for sharing some resources which hitherto have had separate funding (e.g. clinical audit, complaints, risk management, etc.).

Table 3.4 Benefits of clinical governance: the vision for the next five years[3]
From *Clinical governance: Quality in the new NHS*

Areas of change	Benefits of change
A new culture in NHS organisations	Open and participative, and can demonstrate this both internally and to external bodies such as the Regional Office of the NHS Executive and the Commission for Health Improvement
	Able to demonstrate a commitment to quality, shared by staff and managers, and supported by clearly identified resources, both human and financial. These resources are part of an agreed development and implementation plan and their use is reviewed by the Board as part of their discussions on clinical governance
	Working routinely with patients, user, carers and the public
	An ethos of multidisciplinary teams working at all levels of the organisation
	Informed and underpinned by education and research activities which are focused on the needs of the organisation and improving the quality of services
	Regular Board level discussion of the big quality issues for the organisation and strong leadership from the top
	Good use of information to plan and assess progress
Inequity and variability	Unjustifiable variations in the quality of care provided (including outcomes, access, and appropriateness) between services in different areas are reduced through quality improvement
	NHS organisations are working to ensure that they are making progress against recognised benchmarks
Involving users and carers	An organisation-wide strategy for involving patients, users, carers and the public, including strategic plans for communicating with them
	Designated senior individual to oversee patient, user, carer and public involvement strategy
	User representatives on clinical governance committee/groups

	Use of involvement methodologies, e.g. patient panels, focus groups
	Training and education for all individuals on effective patient, user, carer and public involvement
Sharing of good practice	Evidence that individuals and organisations are actively learning from others, for example by actively seeking out and making use of examples of good practice and of the ways in which particular issues have been tackled elsewhere
	Wasteful duplication of effort is minimised
Detecting and dealing with poor performance and adverse events	Poor performance is the concern of all clinical and managerial staff
	Clear mechanisms for the identification and management of poorly performing clinicians to voice their concerns about performance of their colleagues (taking account of new national policies and procedures
	Poor performance procedures aim to identify practice as it begins to slip, and proactively to support and develop clinical staff, enabling sustained improvements in the vast majority of cases without risk to the quality of patient care.

The concept of stakeholders

As any change affects both individuals and groups within the team or an organisation, and the way they work, it is vital to know from which quarters resistance or support of the proposed change will come. It is here that the concept of 'stakeholders' needs be elucidated.

Stakeholders are individuals and groups who are affected by change and are capable of influencing it either positively or negatively. There are three main types of stakeholders:[10]

- Key individuals within an organisation or team
- Key groups or 'tribes' within an organisation or team
- Key external individuals and influences.

It is important to identify the less obvious stakeholders in addition to the more obvious groups who may influence the process of change when examining all three levels. The box indicates an example:

In the immediate situation (for example, a mental health team) the stakeholders could include:
- Psychiatric nurses
- Psychiatrists (junior and senior doctors)
- Professions allied to medicine (e.g. occupational therapists)
- Psychologists
- Non-clinical staff
- Managers
- Patients and their carers
- Social worker attached to the team
- Voluntary sector organisations.

For wider scale changes, other stakeholders need to be considered, for example:[10]
- Trade unions
- Staff organisations
- Professional and/or statutory groups
- Local politicians
- National politicians
- Competitors – e.g. other similar services
- Local 'experts' – e.g. support staff such as IT or human resources
- Unrepresented staff.

Each group may see any proposed change very differently, for a number of reasons (see Figure 3.3) and stakeholders will vary in their ability to influence change, depending on the source of their power.

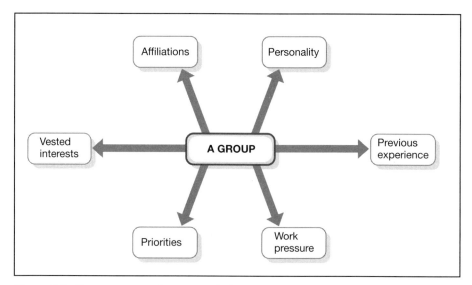

Figure 3.3 Group response to proposed change

Identification and reduction of resistance to change

People react in different ways to proposed change. This is true of a change in life generally (e.g. a new job, moving house, having a baby and so on) and to changes in the work setting (learning how to assess clinical risk, getting feedback from patients, acquiring new clinical skills etc.). Some may welcome a different approach to working, whilst others may find this new position very threatening. Some of the factors facilitating change, and indeed those opposing change, can be easily identified; others require in-depth analysis.

There are some people who do not see the need for change: they consider the way they are currently working to be the best method they know. A case of a clash of personalities may be at the root of the opposition to change.

There are systems for analysing these types of problems in a logical manner. The usual method is called a 'force field analysis' and it is a process by which the influences, or 'forces', are identified in order to facilitate the desired change. A social scientist called Kurt Lewin[11] first proposed that no situation is entirely immovable; that the forces that define a situation are fluid, rather than fixed, and can be influenced. This is similar to a concept in physics which states that when a body is at rest the sum of all the forces acting upon it is zero. Lewin applied this theory to human factors. The premise is that any stable social situation is, in reality, in a state of 'dynamic tension', created by conflicts. The forces supporting and pushing for change (the driving forces) are equally matched by the forces pushing against the change (the restraining forces).

Change, therefore, can be achieved by strengthening (or adding to) the driving forces, or by weakening (or eliminating) the restraining forces. A successful long-term change will occur if the restraining forces are weakened or eliminated. Strengthening the driving forces would result in forcing through change, causing tension or unintentional sabotage.

The force field analysis involves four steps:

Step one

Identification of the desired change. In the case of clinical governance, which is a complex, all-encompassing change, it is probably easier to break it down into more specific changes with clear steps – for example, which areas need to be prioritised, or which processes can be amalgamated (e.g. clinical audit, risk management and care pathways).

Step two

Identification of existing forces that can facilitate the changes specified in step one, and of those that are preventing it or inhibiting it. These forces may be societal factors, other external factors (e.g. government policy), specific groups (e.g. clinicians, managers etc.), or individual people (e.g. the Medical Director, the PCT clinical governance lead). Figures 3.4 and 3.5 illustrate these forces.

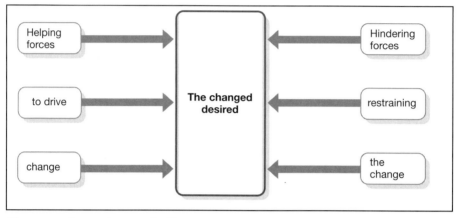

Figure 3.4 Forces that can facilitate change

Following an audit which has demonstrated a lack of knowledge concerning the essential procedures of cardiopulmonary resuscitation to be applied when faced with an unconscious person in the street, a doctor has the task of persuading her colleagues to attend a basic resuscitation course to remedy the situation. The diagram below shows a partially completed force field analysis to illustrate the possible forces for and against the uptake of this recommendation.

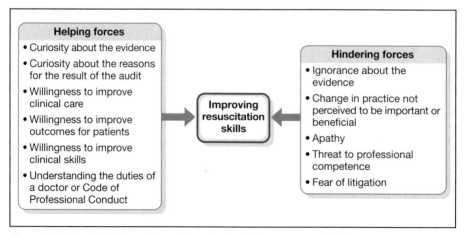

Figure 3.5 Possible forces for and against uptake recommendations

Once the opposing forces have been identified, their relative strengths should be determined. This can be represented diagrammatically by labelling each arrow with the force identified and illustrating the strength of that force by the length or thickness of each arrow. So, for example, if the strength of one force is considered to be twice the size of another, that could be reflected in the longer or thicker arrow representing that force. This can also help the decision as to which forces are the critical ones and so require extra attention.

Step three

This step is about what to do next with the information gleaned during this process. The aim is to change the intensity of the critical or major forces that have been identified in stage two and so reduce the problem. Three options are available to facilitate this change:

● Reduce the restraining or hindering forces
● Increase the driving or helping forces
● Achieve a combination of both.

Beginning with the forces that are preventing or inhibiting change, each one should be taken in turn, examined, and a decision made as to whether anything can be done to reduce the strength of that force. If so, then what should the action be? The more specific the action, the more successful the outcome. The helping forces should be examined in a similar manner, and a decision made as to how each one could be enhanced, if possible. Often it is a combination of both actions that achieves the desired change.

Step four

In the last stage of the process, an assessment should be made of the whole picture as identified in the last three steps and the most feasible actions considered. This is the beginning of the action plan for achieving the desired changes. A time scale is essential. It is helpful to involve the whole team in this action planning process.

Although force field analysis can be perceived as a laborious process, it has been shown to work.

Resistance quadrants[9]

In some instances, there may need to be a further assessment of people's reaction to change, particularly of those who provide resistance to the new ideas. Resistance to change is a combination of covert or overt actions with either conscious or unconscious actions as illustrated in Figure 3.6.

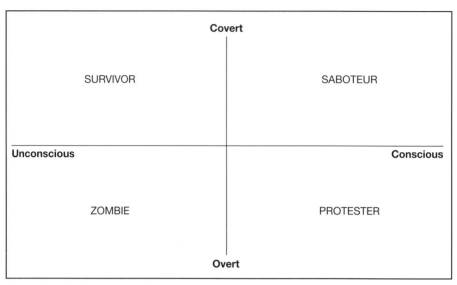

Figure 3.6 Resistance quadrants

- The covert and conscious resistor (saboteur) pretends to support change but in reality does nothing and may actively work against the change.
- The covert and unconscious resistor (survivor) does not realise he is undermining change; for example, he does not realise that he is failing to meet targets or understand the implications of his behaviour.
- The overt and unconscious resistor (zombie) is an extreme case of a survivor. He is so accustomed to acting in a certain way that he is unable to change. He needs constant reminding to change his behaviour.
- The overt and conscious resistor (protestor) is 'a pain in the neck'. He seems to enjoy pointing out the failings of the change. However, he helps to protect against rash change and is the easiest and most interesting person to change in the short term.

Below is a list of some tried and tested ways of reducing resistance to change.

- Allow everyone involved in the planning of the change to participate if they want to.
- Describe clearly the picture of the change.
- Communicate information about the change in practice desired to the fullest possible extent, and continue to keep people updated on the situation. Here, it is particularly important that there is provision of some evidence to support the change in clinical practice that is being negotiated.

- Break down any big changes into smaller, more manageable steps if necessary.
- Reduce the potential for any surprises.
- Clarify any new roles colleagues are expected to assume.
- Provide positive reinforcement for competence – it is important to let people know they can do it.
- Help people feel compensated for the extra time and energy it requires.

Power net analysis

Anyone who works in an organisation, whether a hospital, general practice or part of a community team, will know that in order to get things done there needs to be an awareness and understanding of organisational power and politics. Identifying who will help and who will hinder, why specific events occur and what will influence people to support the aims indicated will go a long way towards achieving the objective of a change in behaviour – and hence attitude and clinical practice.

The exercise of power involves person X influencing person Y to do what X wants. If the question is asked: Why will Y do what X wants?, the answer indicates the level of the power of X. While X can be seen to have sources of power to influence Y, Y usually also has some power, albeit not so obvious. Politics is rarely a one-way system, and it can shift radically over time as things change.

The types and sources of power are complex and often overlap to a large degree. They are also subject to issues of prior inequality between people – particularly in relation to groups who are usually excluded from the decision-making process. People in the work situation may have power according to their attributes of sex, race, physical ability or disability, class, education, age and sexuality. Their power will also be determined by the following factors:[12]

- Formal authority – this is the right of an individual to make decisions bestowed by higher management and/or on the individual's specific role in the organisation. The authority obviously depends on other people's acceptance of that individual's right to exercise this action. It is seldom sufficient on its own and is usually found in conjunction with one or more of the other types or sources of power.
- Expertise – this is technical knowledge and skills, usually acquired through professional training outside the organisation. The more exclusive the expertise and the more useful it is seen to be in the organisation, the more power it confers on that individual.
- Resources – this is the control of physical, financial or information

resources. It is possible for people in relatively low positions in the hierarchy to have considerable power over resources. The pattern tends to be that most power goes to those who control the most valued resources, particularly money and information. People recognise that information is one of the most important political resources, and it requires attention to informal as well as formal channels in order to manage its power.

- Personal attributes – this is the ability to persuade others and to build successfully on good working relationships and networking. This is very much dependent on personal flair as well as on the skills gained through experience, training and conscious practice.
- Gatekeeping – this is the control of access to people, information, resources and decision-makers. This particular barrier or stopping power can be wielded by anyone in the organisation, and can be especially negative or destructive. In some instances, gatekeeping and control of resources reside in the same individual.

The power situation of an individual can be summarised by the drawing of a power net, which can show the relationships with others higher or lower in the hierarchy of an organisation or team and inside and outside the organisation.

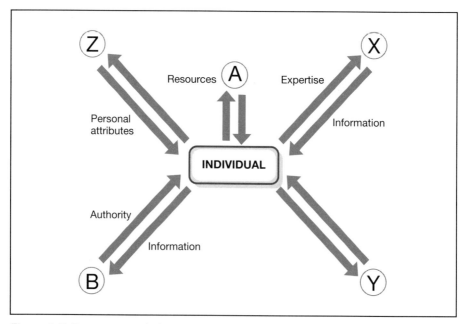

Figure 3.7 Power net analysis

Figure 3.7 shows how the relationships can be illustrated between an individual and others. A number of relationships are shown.

- The individual and person X – this could be the relationship between two colleagues (e.g. physiotherapists) of similar ability and experience. Person X has specific expertise in the management of asthma due to specialist training undertaken in the past; however, this is out of date. The individual at the centre could have the advantage in that their knowledge of a particular aspect of care (e.g. specific techniques in the management of chronic asthma) is based on the latest evidence through the effort of their own research.
- The individual and person Z – this could be the relationship between a doctor and a business development manager. Here the relationship is good. Person Z has confidence in the doctor's abilities to carry out high quality clinical work, and is willing to offer some extra resources to help (e.g. some administrative support, some funding for clinical audit or risk management, help with engaging other stakeholders etc.).
- The individual and person B – this could be the relationship between a doctor and a nurse. The individual (the doctor) will assume authority because of specialist skills or knowledge in the area of the management of patients with, for example asthma. Person B will, in return, have some influence on the doctor, for example, having critically appraised a key research paper on a specific aspect of asthma management. The doctor may not have been aware of the paper.

Building a commitment to change clinical practice

The techniques described above help in the analysis of people's attitudes, motivations and spheres of influence. However, sometimes a further assessment is required, particularly if robust arguments need to be formulated in order to convince others to take up and implement the challenge that the key changes of clinical governance present.

In this circumstance a SWOT analysis is helpful. SWOT stands for Strengths, Weaknesses, Opportunities and Threats. This technique, which was developed at Harvard Business School, and is often used in a marketing context, is used frequently in NHS organisations to achieve change. A SWOT analysis helps clarify the larger picture around the circumstances of change and aids the formulation of arguments. The process is often illustrated in the format set out in Figure 3.8.

STRENGTHS	WEAKNESSES
OPPORTUNITIES	THREATS

Figure 3.8 SWOT analysis

The strengths and weaknesses relate to the internal environment of the organisation or team; for example, the situation of an individual having to introduce the change. The opportunities and threats are concerned with the external environment; for example, the latest government initiative. They are usually factors over which an organisation or team have little or no control. Something perceived as a threat can be turned into an opportunity – for example, the process of clinical governance can act as a trigger for improvement and facilitate a re-examination of clinical practices.

A SWOT analysis works best when the participants (representatives of the team or organisation, or relevant stakeholders) allow their thoughts to fly freely and a note is made of anything and everything that comes to mind when considering the situation, no matter how bizarre it may seem. The ideas created from this process can be ordered later when the flow of thoughts has come to an end, and a clear list can be written down. This method of 'brainstorming' frequently generates ideas and actions in a broader context which other approaches could otherwise curb.

A useful note to consider when drawing up a SWOT analysis is to address each heading separately and list the issues under those different headings. It is essential to keep the lists separate so that the issues are not mixed up together. It is possible for some items to appear in two lists (e.g. something may be both a threat and a potential opportunity).

It is important to specify how each of the items identified are strengths, weaknesses, opportunities and threats. For example putting 'your manager colleagues' under the threat banner does not describe why they are a threat. Is it their strong views on how clinical governance should be imposed in the organisation, or their approach of working with specific medical colleagues to implement the process?

The outcome of a SWOT analysis is to identify the main issues that need to be addressed as a clear action plan. There will be elements in the SWOT analysis that cannot be influenced, and this is to be expected. An action plan is likely to be successful if it concentrates on the areas (people and actions) that can be influenced.

A way of focusing on the analysis is to ask the following questions:[12]

- What are the main issues I must address?
- What must I do to achieve the change in practice I want?
- What strengths in my practice should I build on or exploit?
- What weaknesses in my practice must I tackle?
- What opportunities should I develop?
- What threats must I counteract or minimise?

Using these questions will guide the development of the main aims that should be tackled to obtain the required change in clinical practice.

Highlighting deficiencies in colleagues' clinical practice is both threatening to the recipients and unpleasant to the initiator. It may be perceived as criticism, and will close the doors on any potential constructive dialogue.

One of the ways in which this can be made less threatening is through the use of clinical audit or care pathways (see Chapter 5). When performed well, this is a good motivator in changing behaviour as the information is perceived to be impartial. All good health professionals are interested in the results of the health care they provide to patients; therefore, checking the quality of care against agreed standards using audit generates lively and constructive discussion about current clinical practice.

In some circumstances there may be a need for a further analysis of the issues highlighted by the SWOT process – in particular, some of the key external influences on the organisation (i.e. the opportunities and threats) that will drive change in a specific direction. These can be examined by the use of a PESTELI analysis – looking at political, economic, social, technological, ecological, legal and industry influences. Table 3.5 shows some of the major external influences on an organisation with regards to clinical governance. The questions that relate to these factors are:

- which of these are the most important currently?
- which of these are important in the next few years?

Differentiating the factors that have a long-term influence from those that may be ephemeral will make best use of the effort involved in achieving change.

Table 3.5 PESTELI analysis of clinical governance

Political
- government to promote quality of care
- various government initiatives for change e.g. PCTs, walk-in clinics, whole systems approaches
- government strategies (e.g. clinical governance, Our Healthier Nation etc.)

Economic
- overall investment in health by government – how this is targeted
- priority setting
- general economic climate – impact on health

Social
- ageing population
- lifestyle changes
- public expectations of health care
- change in working practices

Technological
- new interventions and technologies
- telemedicine
- research evidence – effect on NHS R&D strategy

Ecological
- disposal of clinical waste
- using disposable instruments

Legal
- Human Rights Act
- consent procedures

Industry analysis
- attractiveness of the NHS to potential employees

These approaches may not work in all situations – for example, the drawing up of guidelines for local implementation. In these sorts of occasions another approach is necessary.

Commitment charts

The identification of the relevant stakeholders who may help or hinder the achievement of change and of their potential positive participation in working out in detail the precise action plan required are important steps. However, the action plan will only actually work if the support and commitment from these individuals (and others who may be affected) is obtained. One way of identifying people's commitment to change is to follow these steps:[13]

- List the key stakeholders who are required to support the change

- Select from the list the stakeholders whose support is essential; they are the 'critical mass' of support
- Assess the current level of commitment from each individual within this 'critical mass'
- For each individual, assess what the desired future level of commitment should be for the successful implementation of the proposed change. This step should highlight who should be involved.

Showing this process diagrammatically can help to clarify the level of commitment and the change required (Table 3.6). The level of commitment can be judged using the following scale for each individual:

No commitment	Likely to oppose the change
Let it happen	Will not oppose the initiative but will not actively support it
Help it happen	Must provide resource (time or equipment)
Make it happen	Must be actively involved and willing to lead

Table 3.6 Commitment chart

Key stakeholders	No commitment	Let it happen	Help it happen	Make it happen
1		⊠ →	→	○
2				⊠ ○
3		⊠ →	○	
4	⊠ →	○		
5			⊠ ○	
6		⊠ →	→	○
7			⊠ →	○
8		⊠ ○		
9	⊠ →	→	○	
10			○	← ⊠

Key: ○ = Required level of commitment   ⊠ = Current level of commitment

Table 3.6 illustrates how a person's current position and where they need to be for the change to occur can be shown. The difference between the two is a rough measure of the work which may need to be done in order to obtain the necessary commitment from key the stakeholders. In this chart, stakeholders 5 and 7 hold the required position and stakeholders 1 and 6 have the furthest to move. Stakeholder 10 represents an individual who, although committed, may adversely affect the process if they were involved – for example, their interpersonal skills may put off others whose commitment is vital. Stakeholder 2 is most likely to act as a 'champion for change' as their current and required level of commitment coincide, and fall in the 'making it happen' column. It is helpful if that champion has the respect of others within the team or organisation, and if the remaining stakeholders are likely to be willing to follow their lead.

Responsibilities

A method for ensuring a successful change in the way people work is to look at the responsibilities of those involved in the change process. The drawing up of a responsibility chart will illustrate the level of responsibility the key people have for each task according to the following five categories:[14]

A = Approve, powers of approval and veto
R = Responsible for action and delivery once approval has been given
P = Provide resources
I = To be kept Informed, but otherwise not involved
C = To be Consulted before decisions are taken

It is important to have only one person responsible for a particular task. If more than one person is responsible, then the task should be divided into clear distinct parts with a person assigned to each part. Alternatively, the responsibility should be raised to a more senior management level so that one person has overall responsibility. It is also helpful to keep the approval responsibility to one person, otherwise the process may be slowed down.

Issues for consideration

Consider your organisation or team.

- What are the opportunities and threats for implementing clinical governance?
- How can the major barriers be overcome?
- Who are the 'champions for change'?

The role of the strategic health authority in clinical governance

The various management techniques discussed above can be used in most situations to obtain a change in behaviour and hence increase the chances of developing the clinical governance process in a positive way. Individual NHS organisations are required to set up clinical governance systems as discussed in the previous chapter; however, there is a need for an overall co-ordination of the process within a defined geographical area. Strategic health authorities are in a position to provide this type of leadership and facilitation across a number of NHS bodies within their jurisdiction, through performance management processes.

In the previous chapter we have seen that all NHS bodies are accountable for the health care they purchase and deliver under the statutory duty of corporate governance, which incorporates clinical governance.

In its discussion document in 1999, the London region identified six areas in which health authorities would require accountability for clinical quality and for co-ordinating the process with partners.[15] The rationale here was that although health authorities did not directly provide clinical care, they did have functions which involved clinical matters. Since the establishment of strategic health authorities, many of the more 'hands on' health authority functions have been delegated to other organisations such as PCTs.

Despite the changing picture, the six areas of accountability identified by the London region are still applicable.

- Programmes of health care for diseases (e.g. diabetic care), screening (e.g. cervical cancer) and prevention (e.g. smoking prevention as a means of reducing lung cancer and coronary heart disease)
- Provider providence of clinical governance by, for example, local trusts and primary care trusts
- Intersectoral services requiring close collaboration between health and other public services such as social services
- Systems such as information and infrastructure (e.g. training collaboration) on which clinical governance is dependent
- Statutory and formal responsibilities of a clinical nature
- The public health function.

Programmes of health care

Disease programmes
The setting and monitoring of the standards of care to patients provided by

one trust or PCT is the responsibility of that NHS organisation. If the patient care is provided by more than one organisation, the Health Authority is well placed to ensure that approaches to the standards are compatible, consistent and agreed jointly with relevant stakeholders and clinicians. The types of diseases requiring this approach are those that:

- exist across a number of trusts or across primary and secondary care
- are highly complex
- have treatments based on good evidence of effectiveness
- have treatments that are expected to reduce substantially the burden of disease
- have a population perspective.

Some examples include hypertension, maternity care, asthma and severe mental illness. The National Service Frameworks require district-wide quality standards.

Screening programmes

These programmes require the measurement of performance against national and/or locally agreed standards and examples include breast cancer, neonatal services, cervical cancer and child health screening.

Preventive programmes

Examples include accident prevention, vaccination and immunisation, alcohol and drug education, anti-smoking campaigns, and nutrition and good parenting programmes.

Provider providence

Although each NHS organisation is responsible for its own internal clinical governance arrangements and accountabilities, the strategic health authority needs to ensure that each local organisation is fulfilling its responsibilities in this area. This is done through a mechanism of performance agreements with individual PCTs and NHS trusts.[16]

Primary care

In the early stages of PCG development, the health authority concentrated on ensuring that satisfactory arrangements were in place in each general practice. As PCGs developed into primary care trusts, the monitoring of standard setting and performance review for primary care services was transferred to PCTs.

Secondary care

Initially the health authority assessed the performance of their local trusts through reports on clinical audit, clinical risk management, clinical effectiveness, quality assurance, staff and organisational development and through an assessment of satisfactory responses to national audit reports such as the National Confidential Enquiries, the National Service Framework standards and NICE guidelines. As PCTs began to be established this function was delegated to them.

Intersectoral services

A number of patient services are dependent on organisations outside the NHS, such as social services (for child protection), Mental Health Act workers, community care and continuing care. Other agencies include the criminal justice system (for drug addiction, mental health and prisoners' specific health needs such as AIDS, drug addiction and sexually transmitted diseases) and local authorities for housing and environmental matters. Here, a balance needs to be struck between conflicting interests.

Taking the example of environmental issues, there may be conflicts with health matters – for example, better insulation of households saves energy but increases the prevalence of dust mites which are a major contributing factor for childhood asthma and allergy. Similarly, the burning of wood (a renewable source of energy) is encouraged, and the use of diesel vehicles is promoted because of their relatively low emissions of carbon dioxide; however, both lead to an increased emissions of fine particles which have been associated with adverse health effects at levels below current air quality guidelines.

Working across sectors requires plans and policies to be agreed at the operational level and that joint standard setting, monitoring, audit and training occur. This should be reflected in the local delivery plans.

Health systems (information and community infrastructure)

In order to assess performance, it is necessary to compare like with like and to collect compatible information across different health sectors (e.g. secondary and primary care).

Another important support to the development of a consistent approach to clinical governance and the maintenance of high quality care is multidisciplinary training and education. Successful implementation is more likely if there is collaboration between local NHS organisations, training institutions (e.g. the universities) and education consortia than if developed in isolation. The health authority was well placed to facilitate such partnership working. This function is being taken over by workforce development confederations.

These topics will be developed further in Chapter 7.

Statutory and formal responsibilities of a clinical nature

These include roles such as the supervision of midwives and child protection. These areas demand clinical skills at a high level. The professionals involved need to set appropriate standards and measure their performance against them.

Assessing the quality component of service agreements requires professional involvement, particularly the clinical effectiveness of purchasing decisions. Robust evidence to support the commissioning or funding of specific interventions and not others is essential in the decisions to purchase health care.

The public health function

Public health includes a number of services which can be considered in the same way as services requiring clinical standard setting and monitoring. Examples are infectious diseases, environmental hazard investigation, emergency planning and Section 47 work. There are other public health functions, such as needs assessment, planning and epidemiological evaluation of services which could be viewed either as clinical or managerial in nature. The different public health functions are spread across different organisations such as PCTs, strategic health authorities and the regional offices of government.[16]

TABLE 3.7 Clinical governance in Berkshire[17]

In Berkshire there are two strategies, one for clinical care (clinical effectiveness and clinical governance) and the other for evidence-based commissioning, policy and management.
N.B. Although this was originally designed with a health authority in mind, the principles could apply to PCTs.

Objective 1: to promote clinical effectiveness and clinical governance across the whole of Berkshire

Inform	The health authority will share information on clinical effectiveness and clinical governance by the following: • commission a Berkshire-wide NHS website with a page that provides information on clinical topics

- issue a clinical quality newspaper with a paper version of the framework above and updates from the National Institute for Clinical Excellence – NICE, regional office etc.
- have a 'Chief Knowledge Officer' for Berkshire (see Chapter 4)
- development education and training such as the critical appraisal skills programme – CASP (see Chapter 4)
- have a strategic group to provide direction to clinical governance
- promote closer links with local universities

Change   Change the health authority to:
- implement a 'bottom up' approach to clinical effectiveness reviews
- implement the National Service Frameworks (NSFs)

Monitor   The health authority will:
- monitor the development of clinical governance systems
- ensure that good news about improved practice is disseminated in addition to bad news about poorly performing practitioners
- develop shared achievable targets

Objective 2: to successfully support plans to implement clinical effectiveness and clinical governance programmes in trusts

Inform   The health authority will support trusts in:
- clinical effectiveness education
- supporting CASP initiatives
- clinical governance support systems
- NSF implementation
- NICE guidelines

The health authority will also support trusts in:
- sharing information, thereby preventing duplication of effort
- sharing problems, successes and failures

Change   The health authority will help trusts:
- to prioritise clinical effectiveness reviews/topics
- by providing resources – implementing clinical and cost effectiveness programmes may mean high transition costs (e.g. leg ulcer treatment)

Monitor   The health authority will:
- monitor systems in place for clinical effectiveness

Objective 3: to develop clinical effectiveness and clinical governance programmes in PCGs

Inform   The health authority will support PCGs by:
- developing education (e.g. CASP), clinical effectiveness, clinical governance processes and other useful tools (e.g. needs assessments and priority setting)

- information/ knowledge strategies (e.g. develop electronic links to all practices, web sites etc.)

Change   The health authority will work:
- closely with the primary care leads and local medical committee to develop clinical governance
- to develop budget plans for clinical governance and clinical effectiveness
- to promote the concept of a 'Chief Knowledge Officer'
- the primary care clinical audit group will develop appropriate methods of clinical audit to support clinical governance

Monitor   The health authority will ensure that systems are in place for:
- audit of clinical governance and clinical effectiveness
- developing clinical effectiveness topics
- reviews of clinical governance processes with PCG boards

Evidence-based commissioning, policy and management

The Health Authority will use evidence for effectiveness of health care to support its decisions for commissioning and for advice to PCGs. An evidence-based needs-led policy function will be set up to provide advice on:
- new emerging technologies, drugs and services
- needs assessment
- evidence-based support/clinical effectiveness.

The National Service Frameworks form the basis of some of the developments listed above.

(From Berkshire Health Authority)

Success criteria in clinical governance

Once the change has been achieved and clinical governance is running smoothly in an NHS organisation, there needs to be a process of monitoring the progress to ensure that systems are functioning appropriately. The measures used should be consistent, whether the institution being assessed is a primary care trust, health authority or NHS trust.

A suggested set of success criteria has been produced by the London Regional Office of the NHS Executive, which include both process and outcome measures.[18] They are:

- Appropriate cultural/environmental conditions
- Staff and organisational development
- General overview and bringing together
- Clinical audit

- Clinical risk management
- Clinical effectiveness
- Quality assurance.

Each of these has a number of specific measures attached to them and the full list is in the toolkit at the end of this book. The measures reflect the principles of clinical governance.

In this chapter the emphasis has been on the approach to change and how that can be achieved. It is clear that any number of change management techniques can be used to identify the opportunities for implementing the changes required by clinical governance. The key process is to ensure that the circumstances within which change is to occur have been analysed thoroughly, that the key stakeholders have been identified and that there is a critical mass of commitment supporting the change.

In terms of key roles, each NHS organisation is responsible for setting up its own clinical governance systems, and health authorities, with their larger population perspectives, have an important function in co-ordinating the overall development and monitoring of the process.

References

1. The Secretary of State for Health 1998 A first class service: quality in the new NHS. NHS Executive, London
2. Royal College of Nursing, RCN Information 1998 Guidance for nurses on clinical governance. Royal College of Nursing Institute, London
3. Department of Health 1999 Clinical governance: quality in the new NHS. Health Service Circular 1999/065
4. Maslow A 1970 A theory of motivation. In: Motivation and personality. Harper and Row, New York
5. Armstrong M 1996 A handbook of personnel management practice, 6th edn. Kogan Page, London
6. Hertzberg F 1966 Work and the nature of man. World Publishing Company, Cleveland, Ohio
7. McClelland D C 1961 The achieving society. Van Nostrand, New York
8. Vroom V H, Deci E L (eds) 1970 Management and motivation. Penguin, London
9. O'Connor C 1993 The handbook of organisational change. McGraw-Hill, London
10. Meadows S, Gill P, Hearn P et al 1993 The people pack: a step by step guide to getting the best from your workforce. Outset Publishing Limited, St Leonards-on-Sea
11. Lewin K 1947 Frontiers in group dynamics: concept, method and reality in social sciences: social equilibria and social change. Human Relations 1(1): 5-41
12. Marsh S, Macalpine M 1995 Our own capabilities: clinical nurse managers taking a strategic approach to service improvement. King's Fund Publishing, London

13. Barnes P 1995 Managing change. In: Simpson J, Smith R (eds) Management for doctors. BMJ Publishing Group, London
14. Upton T, Brooks B 1995 Managing change in the NHS. Kogan Page, London
15. Department of Health The role of the health authority in clinical governance. http://www.doh.gov.uk/ntro
16. Department of Health 2001 Shifting the balance of power, securing delivery. Department of Health, London
17. Berkshire Clinical Quality Forum 1998 A new strategy for clinical effectiveness and how this supports clinical governance in Berkshire. Berkshire Health Authority, Reading
18. Department of Health A discussion paper on success criteria in clinical governance. http://www.doh.gov.uk/ntro

4

Quality initiatives – the process of clinical effectiveness
Part one: research and development and guideline formation

The quality of clinical care driven by a programme of quality improvement activities within an organisation of any size underpins the principles of clinical governance. The effectiveness of clinical interventions on a patient and the resulting outcome is the cornerstone of the whole process and evidence-based practice provides the support to this.

Although it cannot be disputed that the majority of professionals within the NHS do strive to provide effective care to the best of their ability, the reality is that for one reason or another the care does not necessarily lead to better outcomes for patients.

An illustration of this is the survey by Walshe and Ham[1] on the implementation of clinically effective treatments. In 1996, they sent out a questionnaire to 105 health authorities and 460 trusts in England and Wales, and 71 health authorities and 192 trusts responded. One of the questions asked if clinical practice had changed following the dissemination of the recommendations of three *Effective Healthcare Bulletins* produced by the NHS Centre for Reviews and Dissemination, University of York. The bulletins concerned the management of cataracts (produced in February 1996), in which the recommendation was to increase the proportion of day-case surgery; the management of benign prostatic hyperplasia (December 1995), which recommended substitution of transurethral incision of the prostate for transurethral resection of the prostate as an operation; and the prevention and treatment of pressure sores (October 1995). The findings revealed that the impact of the bulletins was varied (Table 4.1).

Table 4.1 Findings of Walshe and Ham survey[1]		Effective healthcare bulletin		
		Management of cataracts	Management of benign prostatic hyperplasia	Prevention and treatment of pressure sores
Health Authorities (percentage)	Clinical practice has changed	48.3	4.8	8.5
	Clinical practice has not changed	16.7	21.0	13.5
	Not known whether clinical practice has changed	35.0	74.2	78.0
Trusts (percentage)	Clinical practice has changed	48.1	12.1	36.0
	Clinical practice has not changed	34.6	34.5	48.0
	Not known whether clinical practice has changed	17.3	53.4	16.0

The table clearly demonstrates that there has been selective uptake (if any at all) by trusts and health authorities of key clinical recommendations. The study also revealed that access to the information was an important factor in that there were restrictions by trusts' libraries to certain clinical groups (notably non-medical personnel), opening hours were limited, or there were no on-site facilities at all.

Another factor in determining the successful uptake of evidence-based practice is the commitment of an organisation to research and development initiatives. In their survey of 58 health professionals, including doctors, nurses, professionals allied to medicine, psychologists and managers, Eldridge and South[2] found that a positive attitude to research and development within trusts promoted good clinical practice. This was particularly marked in trusts that had longstanding links to academic institutions.

The effective distribution of information within an organisation determines, to some extent, the take up of new research findings. Richardson,[3] in her study, found that trusts and health authorities nominated a wide variety of people to fulfil the function of distributing the *Effective Healthcare Bulletins* produced by York University's NHS Centre for Reviews and Dissemination. Whilst a great proportion of the organisations gave this responsibility to the Chief Executive or another director of the board, several delegated the task to seemingly inappropriate people – such as the personal assistant to the Chief Executive, personnel staff and office managers.

Issues for consideration

● Consider the possible barriers to obtaining appropriate information to improve clinical practice within your organisation. How may they be overcome?

Even in the most forward-thinking organisations, it is unlikely that the information required at a particular point in time will be available immediately to the clinician concerned. It was Muir Gray[4] who highlighted the 'two laws of dissemination':

1. The probability that a disseminated document will arrive on someone's desk the moment it is needed is infinitesimally small
2. The probability that the same document will be found three months later, when it is needed, is even smaller.

Muir Gray then proposed that, given that knowledge needs to be managed by the organisation, there should be someone responsible for this process, the 'chief knowledge officer'. This role of this person is, for example, to look through new reviews produced by the Cochrane Centre and identify that action is required of the board; to ensure that the people responsible for purchasing equipment receive appropriate information; or to ensure that information to patients and carers is evidence-based and comprehensive.

What is clinical effectiveness?

Clinical effectiveness was first officially included on the Department of Health's agenda through the issuing of the guidance *Improving Clinical Effectiveness*[5] and there have been a number of definitions to explain the process.

Although the process of clinical effectiveness is multifaceted and complex, it is possible to break it down into four clearly defined steps:

1. The production of the clinical evidence through primary research and scientific review

2. The production and dissemination of clinical guidelines that are based as much as possible on the evidence available
3. The implementation of evidence-based, cost-effective practice through education, training and change management
4. The assessment of compliance to agreed practice guidance and the evaluation of patient outcomes through quality monitoring processes including clinical audit.

These steps could, in fact, be envisaged as a simple cycle of 'do and review', as clinicians should inform researchers about gaps in knowledge as well as researchers providing the evidence for clinicians to use in their day-to-day practice. The cycle is similar to the audit cycle.

The Department of Health has defined clinical effectiveness as:

The extent to which specific clinical interventions, when deployed in the field for a particular patient or population, do what they are intended to do – i.e. maintain and improve health and secure the greatest possible health gain from available resources.

To be reasonably certain that an intervention has produced health benefits, it needs to be shown to be capable of producing worthwhile benefit (efficacy and cost effectiveness) and has produced that benefit in practice.[6]

Another definition of clinical effectiveness has been produced by the Royal College of Nursing:

The application of the best available knowledge, derived from research, clinical expertise and patient preferences, to achieve optimum processes and outcomes of care for patients.[7]

For an individual clinician, the following checklist of questions can be asked to assess whether a professional is working effectively,[7] as part of life-long learning (see Chapter 7).

- Am I using sound evidence to help me make my clinical decisions or to work up local standards and criteria for best practice?
- Have I considered how I can involve patients and their carers, where appropriate, in making choices about their health care?
- Am I keeping abreast of the latest changes in clinical practice, and how am I doing this?
- How am I approaching the challenge of implementing changes in clinical practice?
- How do I evaluate the care that I am providing?

In the situation of a hectic community caseload, busy ward, outpatient clinic or GP surgery it is sometimes difficult to analyse clinical practice critically.

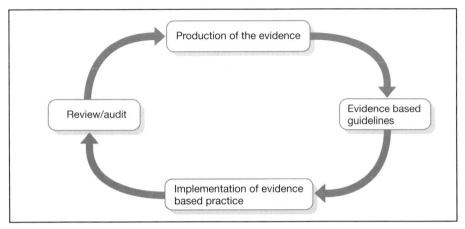

Figure 4.1 Cycle of do and review

The essence of clinical effectiveness is to facilitate this process of evaluation, and the starting point is whether current research has been implemented.

Research and development

Although the NHS was established in 1948 with the aim to provide health care free at the point of delivery, there was no overall perspective or understanding as to how effective this health care was until over 40 years later. In 1991, the first coherent strategy for research and development was produced. Its aim was to 'create a knowledge based health service in which clinical, managerial and policy decisions are based on sound information about research findings and scientific developments. The research and development programme focuses on the needs of the NHS'.[8]

This was soon followed by a report on the support for research in England called *Supporting Research and Development in the NHS*[9] produced by a task force chaired by Professor Anthony Culyer, Professor of Economics at the University of York. The report recommended the introduction of a single funding stream and new arrangements for the allocation and management of support funding for research and development (R&D) including an implementation plan setting out the timetable for securing the new arrangements by 1st April 1998. The recommendations were also applicable to Scotland, Northern Ireland and Wales. The goals were to ensure that all parts of the NHS, including the primary and community care sectors, had equitable access to R&D funding and that those who carried out and supported research justified their claim for funding, in competition with others, and were made accountable for their work.

Most of the NHS funding for R&D comes from the NHS levy, one of five levies on health authority allocations. The R&D levy is held by the NHS Executive. The remainder of the R&D funding covers R&D activity across a number of policy areas, chiefly through the Policy Research Programme (the aim of which is to provide a knowledge base for ministers and officials covering health and social services policy, and central policies directed at the health of the population as a whole) and research undertaken by sponsored non-departmental public bodies such as academic institutions.

The type of projects that the R&D levy is used for are defined as:

- those designed to provide new knowledge
- those whose findings are potentially of value to those facing similar problems elsewhere (i.e. it is generalisable)
- those whose findings are planned to be open to critical examination and accessible to all those who could benefit from them; in other words, for public dissemination.

All the R&D projects are subject to the same principles and assessment criteria (see below). The aim of the R&D strategy is to promote research in all sectors of the NHS – particularly in primary care where this has been poorly developed – and to encourage more multidisciplinary activity.

The principles and assessment criteria for R&D projects[10]

- Quality – according to prevailing professional standards. Not to be used to support unnecessary duplication of R&D effort.
- Ethics – must have received ethical committee approval.
- Relevance, impact and importance – i.e. is 'relevant to health gain in the short, medium or long term and which will contribute to the development and implementation within the NHS of evidence-based practice'. The views of those working in the NHS must be taken into account, and there is a requirement that the R&D evidence has influenced policy and practice within the NHS and that there are links with clinical effectiveness and audit activity.
- Primary care R&D activity is encouraged as it is underdeveloped relative to other sectors in the NHS (this is beginning to change).
- Partnership – working effectively with appropriate partners, including universities, other NHS and academic bodies, service users, carers, local authorities and industry.
- Appropriate disciplinary mix – this is also underdeveloped and needs to be promoted.
- Cost – the R&D funds should be used as efficiently as possible.
- Integration with other NHS activities.
- Management – evidence of effective management of the R&D projects.

Sources of the evidence/information

The evidence for the effectiveness of interventions can be found in research papers. There are many different types of research, some of which are briefly explained below.

Primary research

In primary research, the focus is on patients or populations. The findings are usually published in scientific journals and are written primarily by researchers for other researchers. Primary research is divided into two types: quantitative and qualitative.

Quantitative research

Most scientific research is quantitative, with the emphasis on numbers. Quantitative papers deal with numerical values, a wide range of statistical tests and key statistical concepts such as significance.

Qualitative research

Qualitative research employs a different approach, usually through surveys that are conducted as face-to-face interviews, telephone or written surveys or by focus groups. Interpretation of the findings is subjective.

Systematic reviews

As the primary research base is enormous and increasing rapidly, systematic reviews are the generally accepted method by which evidence can be gathered. The focus of systematic reviews is on reviewing primary research; hence the alternative term, secondary research. The process involves a review of the evidence on a topic that has been systematically identified, appraised and summarised according to predetermined criteria.

There are many sources of evidence available. For the busy or inexperienced clinician or manager, the process of seeking the relevant information can be daunting. However, the National Electronic Library for Health[11] has been set up to guide NHS staff through the maze of information and to simplify the access (see Chapter 7).

Table 4.2 Sources of evidence (from Information for Health[11])

Source	Details
The Cochrane Library	An electronic library, part of the International Cochrane Collaboration, which is regularly updated and is produced by the UK Cochrane Centre in Oxford. Its aims are to develop and maintain systematic, up-to-date reviews of RCTs of all forms of health care, and to make this information readily available to clinicians and other decision-makers at all levels of health care systems.
	There are four databases:
	● The Cochrane Database of Systematic Reviews (CDSR) – a database of systematic reviews of the effects of health care
	● The York Database of Abstracts of Reviews of Effectiveness (DARE) – a database holding abstracts of reviews and of reports by the American College of Physicians Journal Club and health technology agencies all over the world
	● The Cochrane Controlled Trials Register (CCTR) – this holds a bibliography of over 300,000 controlled trials
	● The Cochrane Review Methodology Database (CRMD) – this contains information on randomised control trials, and reviews the strengths and weaknesses of systematic reviews.
Other CD-ROM and on-line searches	Some examples include:
	● MEDLINE – compiled by the National Library of Medicine, this summarises biomedical research literature (including allied health fields, the biological and physical sciences, the humanities and information science as they relate to medicine and health care)
	● EMBASE (Excerpta Medica Database) – covers biomedical literature from 110 countries and has particular strengths in the areas of drugs and toxicology
	● The Cumulative Index to Nursing and Allied Health Literature (CINAHL).
The NHS Centre for Reviews and Dissemination (under the auspices of NICE)	This is based at York University and produces information specifically for the NHS in the form of *Effective Healthcare Bulletins*, Effectiveness Matters and systematic reviews of research evidence.

Epidemiologically based needs assessments	These summarise the health care needs of a population of 250,000 people for specific diseases or population groups.
Local medical/ nursing libraries	These can be found at the local trust/postgraduate centre, and include Royal College of Nursing local libraries.
The National Research Register	This holds information about research and development projects that are currently taking place in, or are of interest to, the NHS.
The National Electronic Library for Health	This is a virtual library, launched in 1999, to provide easy access to research papers and reviews on best current knowledge about health problems, their causes, prevention and treatment (see Chapter 7). It provides information on scientific knowledge to the NHS, ranging from summaries of primary and secondary research evidence to evidence-based guidance to support clinical practice and evidence-based learning.
Journals	There are many journals which publish research (e.g. *British Medical Journal, The Lancet, Evidence-Based Nursing, Journal of Advanced Nursing, Health Trends* etc.).
The Internet	There is a growing number of Internet sites devoted to health matters.

In assessing the robustness of research findings, there is a hierarchy that researchers and clinicians use to indicate the strength, and hence reliability, of the evidence.

Table 4.3 Hierarchy of evidence (from Muir Gray[4])

Type	Strength of evidence
I	Systematic review in which many well-designed randomised controlled trials feature
II	Randomised controlled trial which is well designed and of appropriate size
III	Trials without randomisation or non-experimental study, e.g. cohort or case control studies
IV	Qualitative studies
V	Opinions of respected authorities, based on clinical evidence, descriptive studies or reports of expert committees

Critical appraisal

Having access to the research literature is not enough in itself to decide whether the evidence will be useful. The clinician or manager needs to develop skills in assessing the research. The Critical Appraisal Skills Programme based in Oxford has developed methods for facilitating this. The process takes the reader through four main steps:

● Asking the right question
● Identifying the right research method
● Finding the evidence
● Appraising the evidence.

Access to the Internet is helpful while going through the steps, but it is not essential and many of the learning points can be pulled out direct from the text.

Why do we need critical appraisal?

You may be sceptical on hearing a media report about a new wonder drug or an operation. How can you establish whether or not the treatment is effective? The answer is to go back to the research, and carry out a critical appraisal. Critical appraisal is a very specific skill, and there are critical appraisal tools available which provide a systematic way of assessing the validity and results of a published article, and its usefulness to the local population.

There are many people working in health care who have not had an opportunity to develop these skills during their professional training. Many practitioners therefore need to acquire these skills as part of continuous professional development (see Chapter 7). For those who have had some exposure already, this process could be a useful way of reinforcing knowledge and skills. There are a number of steps in the practice of evidence-based public health or health care. These are set out in Figure 4.2.

Asking the right question

Defining the question is the starting point of evidence-based decision making. The acronym PICO is helpful in developing the question.[12]

Empowering consumers

It is not only practitioners and public health workers who need the skills to find and appraise evidence. The public (as consumers, patients, clients, local people, voluntary groups, pressure groups or advisory groups) need to be partners in the process of care. They need skills to understand the evidence. This is explored further in Chapter 8.

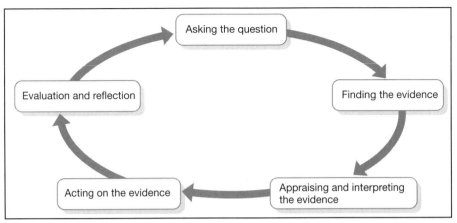

Figure 4.2 The practice of evidence-based public health or health care

P	**I**	**C**	**O**
The problem	**Intervention(s)**	**Comparison(s)**	**Outcome(s)**
The population and the condition you are considering	The intervention you are considering	An alternative intervention with which you would like to compare your intervention	The outcomes you are interested in

Table 4.4 Pico Chart (from Richardson et al[12])

Scenario: Nicotine replacement therapy

Imagine that you are a member of the clinical governance group for your local primary care organisation. The priority for work this year is secondary prevention of cardiovascular disease. One issue that the group considers is support for patients who want to stop smoking. The group debates the place of nicotine replacement therapy. Some members of the group argue that it is useful; others argue that will-power is enough, while still others say that GPs should only recommend nicotine replacement if they can also offer smokers extra support. Someone makes the point that health professionals would need to be trained about all aspects of smoking cessation in order to provide support and advice. You feel that the group's decision might be helped by evidence. You go to your local librarian and together you work on a literature search to find relevant articles, which you are going to critically appraise.

To undertake a literature search you need to be clear of the question you are asking. Before turning over the page try framing a question from the above scenario, using the PICO framework.

Table 4.5 Pico Chart (from Richardson et al[12])

P The problem	I Intervention(s)	C Comparison(s)	O Outcome(s)
Smokers in general practice setting who wish to stop	Nicotine replacement therapy	Placebo or standard treatment	Reduction in numbers who smoke

Our question can now be framed:

In people who smoke, does nicotine replacement therapy, when compared with placebo or with standard treatment, help stop smoking?

Find the right study to answer your question

Clinical governance requires evidence that extends far beyond the issues of effectiveness. Evidence must be accessed to assess best value, risks and safety, to determine acceptability to patients, and to implement research evidence.

There are a number of different types of research methodologies appropriate for these different research questions. No single type of research method is more important than any other. Each has its place in informing decisions. The only truly experimental research is the randomised controlled trial; the other methods are observational.

Table 4.6 The areas of decision making covered by different research studies[12]

Area of decision making assessed	Research study
Prognosis and natural history	Cohort studies
Acceptability to patients	Qualitative research and surveys
The benefits of treatment (also known as effectiveness)	Randomised controlled trials and systematic reviews
Risk, harm and safety	Studies on diagnostic tests and screening, case control and cohort studies
The value of a test, treatment or service	Health economic evaluations
Implementing research evidence	Guidelines and management of change studies

Definitions of different research methods

- A case control study involves the comparison of those with a condition (cases) to those without the condition (controls). The level of exposure to a factor or factors is measured between the two groups and compared.
- A cohort study (also known as a follow-up study, or a longitudinal study) involves the identification of two groups (cohorts), one of which is exposed and the other not exposed to a potential risk factor. These cohorts are followed up in time and the incidence of the outcome in one group compared with the incidence in the other.
- A diagnostic test is any measurement used to identify individuals who could benefit from therapeutic interventions.
- A guideline is a systematically developed statement to assist practitioner and patient decisions about appropriate health care for specific clinical circumstances (see later in the chapter).
- A health economic evaluation is an attempt to express costs and benefits of an intervention in monetary terms.
- A management of change study is a study using qualitative tools to explore the impact of a management intervention.
- A randomised controlled trial is a trial in which subjects are randomly assigned to two groups; an intervention (or experimental) group and a control (or comparison) group. The two groups are following up to see if there are any differences in the outcome of interest. (This is the only truly experimental study – the others involve observation and not experiment.)
- Screening consists of all the steps in a programme, from the identification of the population at risk and the diagnosis of the disease or its precursor in certain individuals, through to the treatment of those individuals.
- A survey or cross-sectional study is one in which information is collected in a planned way in a defined population at one point in time.

For the scenario on nicotine replacement therapy described above, the question is about the benefits of treatment. The study design you would need to look for is a randomised controlled trial, or a systematic review of randomised controlled trials.

Finding the evidence

Accessing evidence

Developments in technology, particularly the Internet, mean that there is access to a huge range of databases. However, if there is no systematic approach to the search, it is easy to waste a large amount of time in seeking information and to end up with only a small proportion of the relevant literature.

This section addresses how access to the evidence can be obtained. It discusses:

- identifying sources of evidence
- building a search strategy
- storing the results
- how the library can help.

Identifying sources of information

Some sources of information are indicated earlier in the chapter and there are references for useful open learning resources (both paper- and computer-based) available at the end of this chapter. The search techniques are applicable to different research methods; however, the other resources mentioned in the references need to be looked up to obtain the relevant checklists.

Evidence is published in a range of sources including books, journals and research reports. For this chapter the focus is on the published literature. There are between 20,000 and 30,000 biomedical journals and 17,000 new biomedical books published annually, which makes the task sound very daunting. Much of the global literature is now captured on databases so that it can be identified and found. Developments in information technology, and in particular the Internet, have linked personal computers with vast databases and have made these easily accessible.

It is easy to waste hours in futile web searches, but a tightly defined question and clarity about which sources to search will make the task easier.

In practice, the search does not need to be so wide every time a question requires an answer. In particular, there are four sources of evidence that can facilitate the search:

- Specialist organisations that are dedicated to summarising research findings and creating databases to aid dissemination – for example, the Cochrane Library (www.update-software.com/cochrane) or Best Evidence (www.bmjpg.com/data/ebm.htm)
- Specialist journals that provide systematic reviews or review high quality primary research, e.g. *Evidence-based Mental Health* or *Clinical Evidence* (www.clinicalevidence.org)
- A range of general and specialised databases, which can be 'searched' using specific techniques to find relevant articles

- The Internet, which offers direct links to organisations that may hold the evidence required.

A detailed description of each of the sources and their advantages and disadvantages is detailed on the CASPFEW website (http://libsun1.jr2.ox.ac.uk/caspfew/sources.html).

This site also has comprehensive, detailed and up-to-date information on sources of evidence, and links to other web-based guides.

Building up a search strategy

In the nicotine replacement therapy scenario described above, we formulated a question:

In people who smoke, does nicotine replacement therapy, when compared with placebo or with standard treatment, help stop smoking?

This sentence has some key words which can be used to structure the search. The local NHS librarian can help in formulating the first search strategy.

Start on the databases of high quality reviews and evidence such as the Cochrane Library and Best Evidence. If those do not come up with relevant studies, then move on to MEDLINE. MEDLINE is the world's largest biomedical database, including nearly 4,000 biomedical journals worldwide. Any search can therefore retrieve several thousand articles. To perform an accurate search, concentrate on specific aspects of the question and this will limit the number of search results to a manageable level. The technique is to start with a broad search (a sensitive search) and then narrow it down (a specific search).

For the question that we are using there are some good references in Cochrane and Best Evidence and it will probably be unnecessary to go any further.

Storing the results

Once the evidence has been found, it makes sense to store it so that it can be easily accessed later.

There are three options:
1. Keeping references with notes in folders or exercise books
2. Maintaining a card index
3. Using personal bibliographic software (reference management software such as ProCite).

Personal bibliographic software (PBS)

This is a class of text retrieval software specifically intended for researchers to manage their personal reference collections. It is designed:
- to handle bibliographic information
- to be friendly/easy to use
- with pre-defined data structures
- with sophisticated search capabilities
- with pre-defined output formats for writing citations (e.g. Harvard, Vancouver formats)
- to produce bibliographies automatically
- so that it is easy to import information from online and CD-ROM databases.

How the library can help

The nearest NHS or higher education library can be a vital ally in the search for evidence. Librarians are trained both to search for evidence and to help others to do it themselves, so it makes sense to tap into this partnership.

In particular, librarians can:

- Help you to find information by:
  - defining boundaries of enquiry i.e. framing the search question
  - talking through information requirements
  - advising on which tools or resources are most appropriate
  - facilitating use of tools by helping you develop search strategies.
- Find information for you by:
  - using their professional expertise to search a wide range of databases and resources
  - liaising with you to obtain a precise profile of information required.
- Provide material for you from:
  - their own stock of journals, reports, books etc.
  - outside sources, via interlibrary loans and other routes.

Many localities have excellent training resources for finding the evidence. If you want to know how to access them, ask your local or regional librarian. Some contacts are set out on the CASPFEW website (http://libsun1.jr2.ox.ac.uk/caspfew).

Appraising the evidence

This section will help you systematically to balance the value and trustworthiness of a study, before deciding whether to act on the evidence. Even papers that have been published in respectable or reputable journals can have inaccurate or confusing conclusions.

There follows a critical appraisal of the systematic review of nicotine replacement therapy that was found as a result of the search above. A copy of the paper, **Silagy C, Mant D, Fowler G, Lodge M. 1994. Meta-analysis of efficacy of nicotine replacement therapies in smoking cessation.** *Lancet* **343: 139–42** appears in the toolkit at the end of the book.

There are some useful hints that will direct you to specific areas and explain why they are so important. Try critically appraising the paper using the 10 questions below before looking at the results of our critical appraisal. Some of the questions can be interpreted in different ways, so you may not agree with the recorded comments all the time. Brief answers are given below, and the learning points are also set out for each question.

The first three questions are screening questions. If it is not possible to give a 'Yes' answer to all three questions, you need to consider whether it is worth carrying on reading the paper.

If you can answer yes to the screening questions, then you can go on to appraise the paper to assess three aspects: its validity, results and usefulness.

Definitions of terms in this appraisal

- Confidence interval (CI): The exact truth is never known, as all trials are carried out on a small sample of the population. CI is a statistical calculation that can help us assess where the truth lies 95% of the time.
- Meta-analysis is a statistical technique that summarises the results of several studies into a single estimate, giving more weight to results from larger studies.
- Numbers needed treat (NNT) is one measure of a treatment's clinical effectiveness. It is the number of people that would have to be treated with a specific intervention (e.g. aspirin for people having a heart attack) to see one additional occurrence of a specific outcome (e.g. prevention of death).
- Odds ratio is a measure of risk, i.e. the likelihood of something happening versus it not happening.
- A quasi-randomised controlled trial is a study in which the investigators lack full control over the allocation and/or the timing of the intervention.

Table 4.7 Critical appraisal skills programme: making sense of evidence about clinical effectiveness (reprinted with permission from Elsevier Science)

10 questions to help you make sense of a review

Silagy C, Mant D, Fowler G, Lodge M. 1994. Meta-analysis* of efficacy of nicotine replacement therapies in smoking cessation. *Lancet*; **343**: 139-42.

General comments

- Three broad issues need to be considered when appraising a review article. Are the results of the review valid? What are the results? Will the results help locally?
- The 10 questions on the following pages are designed to help you think about these issues systematically. The first two questions are screening questions and can be answered quickly. If the answer to both is 'yes', it is worth proceeding with the remaining questions.
- The 10 questions are adapted from: Oxman AD, Guyatt GH et al. 1994. Users' Guides to The Medical Literature. VI: How to use an overview. *JAMA* **272(17)**: 1367-1371.
- The answers on the following pages relate to the paper by Silagy and colleagues in the Lancet about the effectiveness of nicotine replacement therapies in helping people stop smoking. These answers are not necessarily 'right'! They represent the accumulated wisdom from groups attending previous workshops.

A. Are the results of the review valid?

Screening questions

1. Did the review address a clearly focused issue? *HINT: An issue can be 'focused' in terms of* *- the population studied* *- the intervention given* *- the outcomes considered*	The question – is nicotine replacement therapy (NRT) effective in helping people to quit smoking? – is set out in the first sentence of the summary. Population: all smokers wishing to quit, although this is not explicit. Intervention: is defined as NRT, in the forms of gum, patches, spray and inhaler. Outcome: cessation rates, assessed by: a) biochemical confirmation when possible b) sustained quit rates. The follow-up has to be >6 month trials. Side effects of therapy are not assessed in the review due to the variation in reporting of the primary trials. *Learning points*: It is important to be clear about the focus of the question, to confirm that the review is useful to you and will help to inform your question. Unfocused reviews cannot provide you with reliable answers. If it is not focused it is not worth continuing the appraisal.

2. Did the authors look for the appropriate sort of papers?

HINT: The 'best sort of studies' would
- address the review's question
- have an appropriate study design.

Studies included appear to address question asked.

Study design is right because all trials included in the review had to have at least two treatment groups with allocation by a randomised or quasi-randomised method.

Learning points: included studies should closely match up with Question 1 in terms of population, intervention and outcomes. A clear statement of the inclusion criteria makes it less likely that the authors only cite studies that support their prior hypothesis.

Choosing the right sort of study to be included is crucial; as this review is looking at the effectiveness of a treatment, randomised controlled trials should be selected for inclusion.

Is it worth continuing? Yes

Detailed questions

3. Do you think the important, relevant studies were included?

HINT: Look for
- which bibliographic databases were used
- follow up from reference lists
- personal contact with experts
- search for unpublished as well as published studies
- search for non-English language studies

This is an extensive and well-defined search strategy:

7 databases searched; reference lists from clinical trials; conference abstracts; smoking and health bulletins; bibliography of smoking and health; unpublished data – wrote to drug manufacturers.

Learning points: we need to feel confident that the authors looked hard enough to find all studies, both published and unpublished, that met their inclusion criteria. More than one database should be used to maximise the trials found. A thorough search will reduce the risks of:

1) random error which might occur because of small numbers in the trials

2) systematic error from
   - publication bias (this occurs because trials showing no effect or negative effects are often not as likely to be published as those ones favouring a new therapy)
   - retrieval bias (this occurs because trials that are not published in widely read and easy to access journals are not easy to find and include in the review).

4. Did the review's authors do enough to assess the quality of the included studies?

HINT: The authors need to consider the rigour of the studies they have identified. Lack of rigour may affect the studies' results ('All that glisters is not gold!' Merchant of Venice – Act II Scene 7)

All primary studies were RCTs.

Methodological quality was assessed by Chalmers criteria (See reference 9 in the paper).

Specific comments:
Randomisation: randomisation not described in 39 trials

Assessment of outcomes:
- cessation rates – 'strictest criteria' used but not stated what criteria were
- sustained cessation rates used but not stated in how many trials
- blinded validation of smoking status in only 12 trials
- 21 reported smoking status at final follow-up.
- Losses to follow-up defined as continuing smokers.

Learning points: This question asks if the authors assessed the validity of the studies in detail. This should ideally be undertaken by two independent reviewers.

Check: - if the studies were RCTs
   - if the randomisation was robust
   - the completeness of follow-up
   - the intention-to-treat analysis (control of selection bias after entry)
   - blinding and blinding of assessment outcomes.

Studies with weaker designs will be less valid and tend to overestimate the benefits of the treatments.

5. If the results of the review have been combined, was it reasonable to do so?

*HINT: Consider whether
- the results were similar from study to study
- the results of all the included studies are clearly displayed
- the results of the different studies are similar
- the reasons for any variations in results are discussed.*

Consistency in the results of primary studies was high, though trial designs varied in subjects, setting, dosage regimen, measurement of abstinence, losses to follow-up and tapering of the final dose (p.140).

Yes, only 3 trials revealed a negative treatment effect.

Learning points:
It is important to consider whether it was acceptable to combine the primary studies, and the reviewers need to convince us that they were combining like with like.

Look at the graphs and tables, to see if the different studies are finding similar results, or if studies that are using different methodologies are finding similar results.

Think about variations due to populations, intervention/exposure or outcomes, to study methods, or to chance.

B. What are the results?

6. What is the overall result of the review?

HINT: Consider
- if you are clear about the review's 'bottom line' results
- what these are (numerically if appropriate)
- how the results were expressed (NNT, odds ratio etc.)

NRT is an effective intervention, overall odds ratio 1.71.

Numbers needed to treat (NNT) estimates (typically about 30) given for each intervention and stratified for setting and intensity of support.

Learning points:
Is it possible to pull out a 'bottom line' sentence to summarise the findings?
Are they clear and do we understand what they are saying?
See references for further reading and information.

7. How precise are the results?

HINT: Look for confidence interval. This is a statistical calculation that can help us assess where the truth lies 95% of the time.

Precision of overall estimate is high (Confidence interval (CI) 1.56-1.87) because of the large number of subjects. Precision of the estimate for gum and patches is high because of number of trials (subjects). Precision of estimate for inhaler and spray is lower (one trial each).

Learning points: the CI will indicate how precise the results are, as a very wide CI will indicate uncertainty in results. If the CI goes over the line of no difference (i.e. the line of 1) then the results are not statistically significant.

When reading the results, go to the results section looking for each outcome. Sometimes authors will write up the abstract to show their best results, which might not be their main outcomes.

C. Will the results help locally?

Having decided that the research is valid and trustworthy, and what the results are, it is important to establish if the research is transferable to your local population.

8. Can the results be applied to the local population?

HINT: Consider whether
- the patients covered by the review could be sufficiently different to your population to cause concern
- your local setting is likely to differ much from that of the review.

Probably. This review shows NRT to be effective in a wide range of clinical settings.

Benefit seems to be greater for higher dependency levels and those motivated to quit i.e. community volunteers, smoking cessation clinics.

Learning points:
It is important to consider if there are any differences which would make it impossible to apply this to the local population.

9. Were all important outcomes considered?

Main outcome of quitting smoking was reported. Side effects of treatment were not addressed by the review.

Learning points:
Trials are not able to look at all the outcomes in which we may be interested. Consider if the authors have answered their question and whether an important outcome has been missed.

10. Are the benefits worth the harms and costs?

Even if this is not addressed by the review, what do you think?

No information regarding cost and side effects of treatment.

Learning points:
This information is not normally within the trial, but consider yourself what the harms could be and whether these can be outweighed by the benefits. Other research, such as an economic evaluation, might help with the cost implications

Understanding how to appraise a systematic review is an important skill for evidence-based health care. As you become more skilled at critical appraisal, you will find the guides become easier to apply. Many people will interpret the same information in different ways, and the most important message to take away is that professional judgement is essential when interpreting the evidence and making a decision about applying it to your practice.

Critical appraisal of the evidence is a small but very important part of the evidence-based health care jigsaw. Within the decision-making process, many other issues need to be considered – including resources, training, culture, patient acceptability, ethical implications and political agendas.

Returning to our case study

We set out to answer the question:

In people who smoke, does nicotine replacement therapy, when compared with placebo or with standard treatment, help stop smoking?

A systematic review which looked at this question was found.

Our critical appraisal's bottom line was that nicotine replacement therapy is an effective intervention for the primary care group population.

This information is taken back to the clinical governance group. They accept that the evidence is strong enough to make a recommendation but want to see nicotine replacement therapy as part of a comprehensive programme for smoking cessation. The group therefore asks you to find out more about other elements of support to help people stop smoking, including brief advice from GPs, counselling, provision of smoking cessation classes, hypnotherapy and acupuncture. The group wants to see the development of a guideline that can be used by practices within the PCT area.

Very often, one article leads to more questions and the need to find and appraise more evidence. Appraisal is one part of a complex process that results in decision making. Consideration needs to be given to costs, both in terms of human resources and capital; local and national politics; ethical considerations; medico-legal implications and – most important of all – the consumer's values and desires.

Critically appraising other types of studies

Detailed consideration of a systematic review has demonstrated the steps in critically appraising a paper. Other types of studies have different critical appraisal steps. Checklists for systematic reviews, qualitative studies, randomised controlled trials, economic evaluations, diagnostic tests and cohort studies are set out in the toolkit at the end of the book. They are also available to download from the CASP website (www.phru.org/casp).

Clinical guidelines

The use of guidelines in clinical practice has been increasing rapidly, particularly since the 1990s, and they are now a familiar part of routine health care. This has been stimulated by a number of factors, including:

- Rising health care costs, fueled by an increase in patient demand
- More expensive medical technologies

- An ageing population
- Variations in the delivery of health care in hospital and community services
- Geographical variations in health care possibly due to over or under use of services
- The desire of clinicians to provide and of patients to receive the best possible care.

However, there is still some confusion about the role of guidelines and how relevant they are in the day-to-day clinical care of patients. This is exemplified by the use of the terminology referring to the process itself by clinicians.

Different terms have specific meanings, depending on the context in which they are used and the way in which they are perceived by the recipient. Some of the terms that have been used in the past to describe the process include guidelines, protocols, algorithms, practice policies and profiles of care. For example, the term 'protocol' is used extensively in research to describe the process by which the research itself is carried out, an element of which incorporates the idea of guidelines to ensure the researchers follow the same method of working and thus maximise the consistency of the results.

In 1995, Gosfield[13] carried out a survey of hospitals in the United States questioning their use of terminology for guidelines and similar processes. He found that hospitals identified more than 30 different names for initiatives that could qualify for the concept of 'guideline'. The main terms are summarised in Table 4.8.

Table 4.8 Terms used by US hospitals to refer to guidelines

Term used	Percentage of hospitals using the terms identified
Critical paths	42
Practice guidelines/parameters	13
Clinical guidelines	12
Clinical protocols	8
Others, including 'care', 'outcomes', 'paths', 'collaborative', 'tracks', 'processes', 'progressions', 'targets', and 'standards of care'	38

It is not surprising that health care professionals get confused when these different words are used to signify essentially the same process.

Issues for consideration

Consider the use of the different terms signifying the concept of guidelines in your organisation.

● Do different professional groups use the same or different terms?
● What do these terms mean to these groupings?

Nowadays the term that is increasingly used is guidelines. The definition of guidelines that seems to be used frequently by most professionals is the one produced by the Institute of Medicine in the United States. It has defined clinical guidelines as 'systematically developed statements to assist practitioner and patient decisions about appropriate health care for specific clinical circumstances'.[14]

The NHS Executive has developed the definition further and categorises guidelines into two components:[15]

National clinical guidelines

These are the guidelines that have been developed by clinicians and sponsored by the relevant professional body or bodies according to nationally agreed standards. Many institutions have drawn up clinical guidelines.

The National Institute for Clinical Excellence has the task of producing guidelines for health professionals to follow. These guidelines are drawn up taking into consideration the evidence available at the time and a review date is stated to ensure that guidelines are updated regularly.

Institutions that have drawn up guidelines

● The Medical Royal Colleges
● The Royal College of Nursing Institute
● The Royal College of Midwives
● Professional bodies representing professions allied to medicine, e.g. the Chartered Society of Physiotherapists, College of Speech and Language Therapists, and College of Occupational Therapists
● Academic Institutions, e.g. the NHS Centre for Reviews and Dissemination at York University
● Patient Representative Organisations, e.g. Diabetes UK, Action for Sick Children.

Local clinical guidelines

These are guidelines that have been issued at a local level, for example trust, PCT or practice guidelines. These may or may not have been derived from national guidelines. In addition, these are guidelines which have been produced to reflect local needs and priorities where there may not be any national guidelines available. In some cases there may be a number of guidelines for the same condition (e.g. diabetes).

In recent years there has been a proliferation of guidelines not only in the UK but in other countries.[16]

Table 4.9 National guidelines (reprinted with permission of the BMJ Publishing Group[16])	
Country	Number of guidelines
United Kingdom	Over 2000
The Netherlands	Over 70
Finland	Over 700
France	Over 100

In order to avoid duplication of effort, the National Institute for Clinical Excellence has the role of providing a coherent approach to guideline production and maximising the use of professional and academic expertise so that robust, clear and credible information is produced for clinicians to follow.

Benefits and limitations of guidelines

It is important to view guidelines as tools for helping the clinician, in conjunction with the patient, to make the most appropriate decisions on clinical care based on the best available evidence. However, it is not appropriate for clinicians to follow blindly the steps in guidelines, setting aside their clinical expertise and experience without reference to the patient in front of them. Guidelines are there to provide information on the expected outcomes of treatment in the majority of cases. However, patients do vary in their responses to treatment and it is in these situations that clinical acumen takes over from guidelines. Having stated this, guidelines do provide a general reference point for the minimum expected standards of care.

The main benefit of guidelines is to improve the quality of care to patients by improving health outcomes through the promotion of effective interventions and discouraging ineffective care. The result ideally will be to reduce morbidity and mortality and to improve the quality of life.

The principal limitation of guidelines is that the recommendations could be wrong if poorly constructed.

Table 4.10 A summary of benefits and limitations of guidelines to patients, health care professionals and health care systems (reprinted with permission of the BMJ Publishing Group[16])[16]

	Benefits	Limitations
Patients	• improve quality of care • improve health outcomes • improve consistency of care • provide information to patients (e.g. leaflets, videos, audiotapes etc.) • demonstrate available options for treatment to patients • enable patients to influence public policy (e.g. gaps in services, unrecognised health needs, preventive interventions).	• recommendations may be wrong • scientific evidence may be lacking, misleading or misinterpreted • recommendations may be influenced by the opinions, clinical experience and composition of the guideline development group • the patients' needs may not be paramount (e.g. the need to control costs, serve society or protect special interest groups such as doctors, risk managers or politicians) • provide misleading information to patients • adversely affect public policy e.g. reduce access to services.
Health care professionals	• improve the quality of clinical decisions • alert clinicians to interventions not supported by evidence • draw attention to ineffective, dangerous and wasteful practices • form part of a number of quality improvement processes (e.g. care pathways, audit, reminder systems etc.) • highlight areas where there is a gap in the evidence and provide questions for future research.	• promote ineffective, dangerous and wasteful practices • inflexible guidelines may lead to blanket adherence to poor clinical care • conflicting recommendations may confuse practitioners • guidelines may not reflect the complex decision-making required involved in clinical care • could be referred to as citable evidence in medical malpractice • may discourage further research, particularly if an intervention is considered ineffective.

| Health care systems | • improve efficiency and value for money in the delivery of health services (e.g. prescribing costs)
• improve the confidence of the general public in the provision of health services
• free up resources for use in other health care services. | • may compromise operating efficiency or waste limited resources
• may advocate costly or unaffordable interventions or cut into resources needed for more effective services. |

It is important to note that clinicians are expected to follow the guidelines produced by the National Institute for Clinical Excellence and, if this is not done, a careful note should be made in the patient's record explaining why this is so.

Development of guidelines

Many health professionals feel threatened by the concept of guidelines. They believe that the use of guidelines inhibits the clinical freedom of the individual practitioner and does not add to the quality of care of patients. This was the case in the early history of the development of guidelines, when these have been imposed from above with little discussion or modification by the local clinicians. The process is now more sophisticated, and goes through many steps.

- Firstly, guidelines need to be seen as relevant to the day-to-day work of every health care professional – doctors, nurses, professions allied to medicine and so on. The subject of the guideline needs to be seen as an important area to address by all these professionals, and if there is agreement on this with a desire to improve patient care then the stage is set for the next step.
- As we have seen in Chapter 3 it is essential to identify the key stakeholders in the process to maximise the likelihood of a change in practice. Active involvement of all relevant professions, managers and patient representatives is needed in the development of guidelines. This is equally true when bringing national bodies and institutions together for the production of national guidelines, as well as local representatives for the local situation.
- An important aspect of developing guidelines is how these will be disseminated to the health care professionals who will implement them. Past efforts have shown that no single one channel can effect change.

The mechanisms include education and training, meetings, conferences, publications and many other ways of dissemination.

- It is important that local clinicians have an opportunity to review national guidelines. Again, as we have seen in Chapter 3, a force field analysis should identify the indicators for change and the likelihood of success of developing local guidelines. The most practical way of getting the key people together to do this task is through the setting up of a representative group, identified through the stakeholder analysis, to develop the guidelines. The work of the group should address all aspects of the production of the guidelines. This multi-professional group should allow everyone to have their say and ensure that the local perspective is reflected through feedback of comments. This is known as 'local ownership' of the process, when the people involved in drawing up the guidelines are the same as, or represent, those who implement them.

- It is important to reduce, as much as possible, duplication of effort and to use every opportunity to draw on existing work in other parts of the country, in other countries, professional bodies or academic departments. In addition, other quality initiatives happening concurrently locally should be examined for potential incorporation into guidelines.

- There should be clarity on the format in which guidelines are presented – i.e. as a booklet, an A4 laminated sheet, a loose-leaf folder, a poster, a computer programme or a quick reference pocket card. The best way to decide on the format is to determine the target audience and how best to reach them. Examples of presentations are shown below.

Table 4.11 EHH health authority guidelines on oesophageal reflux – lifestyle to improve symptoms to patients[17]

- If you smoke, stop. As well as worsening your reflux problem, smoking can cause fatal heart and lung disease and cancer.
- If you know you are overweight, or if your doctor says that you are, lose weight. Even a few pounds may help.
- Avoid foods or drinks that make your pain or discomfort worse. Things that commonly worsen symptoms include: alcohol, fatty food, spicy food, citrus fruit juice, fizzy drinks (e.g. Cola), coffee, chocolate, mint, tomato, onion.
- Don't drink too much fluid with or just after meals.
- Don't eat late at night or lie down/bend over soon after eating.
- Wear loose clothes. Tight clothes around the waist are likely to worsen your symptoms.
- Raising the head of your bed about 8 inches will often help.

Table 4.12 UK Alcohol Forum guidelines for multidisciplinary team[19]

GUIDELINES

FOR THE MANAGEMENT OF **ALCOHOL PROBLEMS**
IN PRIMARY CARE AND GENERAL PSYCHIATRY

ALCOHOL FORUM UK

ASSESS	EVIDENCE
Elicit patient's own concerns	(See Definition of ratings below)
(presenting problem may not be alcohol)	
Elicit and record	
(1) Consumption over past 3 months	
Typical day's drinking	
Frequency	
Maximum in one day	
(2) Alcohol-related physical, emotional and social problems	
Consider	
(1) Lab investigations	
LFTs, GGT	***GGT (gamma glutamyl transferase) is elevated in about 60% of people drinking >56 units/week (probably less for women). False positives include liver disease of other causes, anticonvulsants.Usually normalises after 2 to 3 weeks of abstinence. (Carbohydrate-deficient transferrin is more discriminatory but not yet in routine use).
MCV	***MCV (mean corpuscular volume) is raised in about 30% of people drinking >56 units/week (probably less for women). Normalises after 1 to 3 months of abstinence.
(2) AUDIT questionnaire	

ADVISE/DISCUSS ←

● **Provide information about health risks**   **In primary care, randomised, controlled studies have shown benefit of GP advice.

● **Patients may not be receptive on first consultation;**
repeated interviews/reviews may be necessary   *** Empathic interview style is more effective than confrontational.

● **Discuss costs and benefits of drinking from patient's perspective**   Motivational interviewing is of proven clinical *** and cost ** effectiveness.

INTERESTED	NOT INTERESTED
● **Agree goal**	● **Sow seeds**

REDUCTION	ABSTINENCE

Indications for advising abstinence

Absolute	Relative	
● **Alcohol-related organ damage**	● **Epilepsy**	***Abstinence should clearly be advised for cirrhosis, dementia or neuropathy.
● **Severe dependence** morning drinking to stop the shakes, previous failed attempts to control drinking	● **Social factors** legal, employment, family	**In particular social situations (e.g. patient presents in crisis, family distress, previous drink-driving offences, imminent threat to job, poor social support) abstinence might well be advised; probable need for assisted withdrawal medication.
● **Significant psychiatric disorders**	● **Other physical problems**	

Definition of evidence ratings
In the preparation of these Guidelines, every effort has been made to reference the content to the best published evidence available. The following notation is used to indicate the extent and quality of the evidence base:
*** Strongly supported by the weight of published evidence.
** Supported by limited published evidence, or balance in sufficient studies is moderately favourable.
* Accepted good practice, although little or no published evidence.

These Guidelines will be reviewed regularly and revised as necessary in the light of significant new published evidence or changes in accepted good practice.

GUIDELINES FOR THE MANAGEMENT OF **ALCOHOL PROBLEMS** IN PRIMARY CARE AND GENERAL PSYCHIATRY

MANAGEMENT PLAN

ABSTINENCE

- Enlist support of family and friends
- Maximise use of local alcohol services (See below)

(1) Achieve abstinence in those drinking
- Plan assisted withdrawal if indicated, at home or in hospital

(2) Maintain abstinence
- Encourage Alcoholics Anonymous

- Consider specific pharmacotherapy (should not be prescribed in the absence of alcohol-focused counselling) There are two specific therapies licensed to help dependent drinkers maintain abstinence in the face of craving:

(i) acamprosate (reduces intensity of and response to cues and triggers to drinking)

(ii) disulfiram (deterrent)

- Initiate active intervention if other psychiatric problems persist e.g. anxiety and depression

- Ongoing support

EVIDENCE

***Outcome is improved if spouse is involved.

*Indications for specialist referral: multiple relapse, concurrent psychiatric illness, potential need for residential rehabilitation.

** AA helps many people and has particular advantage for those who live or work in environments where drinking is encouraged.

Good evidence for acamprosate*** and supervised disulfiram ** in specialised settings with a counselling package but not yet formally tested in general practice.

Naltrexone (not licensed in the U.K. for treating alcohol dependence) is used in some countries to help reduce relapse rates. Currently, there is no published evidence to support its role in 'controlled drinking'.

* Panic and other anxiety disorders common. May respond to antidepressants and/or cognitive-behavioural psychotherapy.
*** Depression responds to antidepressants and/or specific psychotherapy.

REDUCTION

- Review regularly to: Offer encouragement Elicit patient's concerns Ensure self-monitoring of consumption Re-assess costs and benefits of change Help patient recognise and handle situations that might exacerbate drinking
- Consider monitoring GGT, MCV, AUDIT
- Maximise use of local alcohol services

** Brief motivational interviewing and self-control training is effective in non-dependent problem drinkers.

(See below)

RELAPSE

As in many medical and psychiatric disorders, the process of recovery is likely to involve several relapses. Do not give up: carry on with a non-confrontational approach. Useful learning can occur. Consider another form of treatment.

** Patients typically go through the cycle several times before improvement is sustained.

LOCAL SERVICES

Provision of local services is varied. The following may be available: community alcohol service, community alcohol team, alcohol specialist psychiatrist, specialist alcohol unit, CPN with alcohol remit. If social support is insufficient then instigate community care needs assessment through social services. Non-statutory services also play an important role.

Produced by the U.K. Alcohol Forum. Second edition ©2001 Published by Tangent Medical Education.

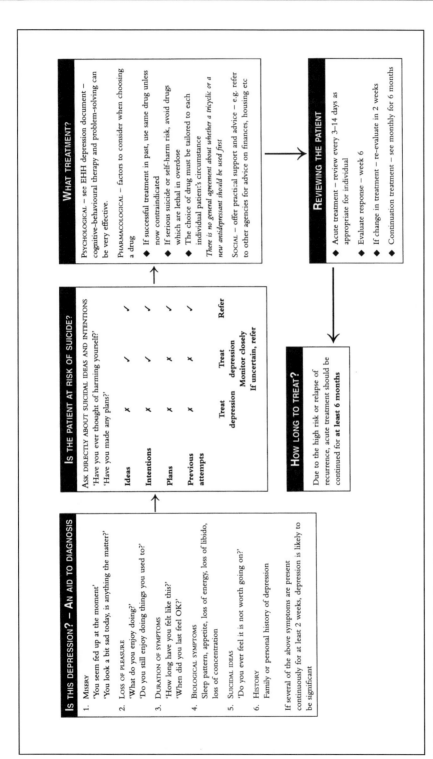

Is this depression? – An aid to diagnosis

1. **Misery**
    'You seem fed up at the moment'
    'You look a bit sad today, is anything the matter?'

2. **Loss of pleasure**
    'What do you enjoy doing?'
    'Do you still enjoy doing things you used to?'

3. **Duration of symptoms**
    'How long have you felt like this?'
    'When did you last feel OK?'

4. **Biological symptoms**
    Sleep pattern, appetite, loss of energy, loss of libido, loss of concentration

5. **Suicidal ideas**
    'Do you ever feel it is not worth going on?'

6. **History**
    Family or personal history of depression

If several of the above symptoms are present continuously for at least 2 weeks, depression is likely to be significant

Is the patient at risk of suicide?

Ask directly about suicidal ideas and intentions
'Have you ever thought of harming yourself?'
'Have you made any plans?'

	Treat depression	Treat depression Monitor closely If uncertain, refer	Refer
Ideas	✗	✓	✓
Intentions	✗	✓	✓
Plans	✗	✗	✓
Previous attempts	✗	✗	✓

How long to treat?

Due to the high risk or relapse or recurrence, acute treatment should be continued for **at least 6 months**

What treatment?

Psychological – see EHH depression document – cognitive-behavioural therapy and problem-solving can be very effective.

Pharmacological – factors to consider when choosing a drug
♦ If successful treatment in past, use same drug unless now contraindicated
♦ If serious suicide or self-harm risk, avoid drugs which are lethal in overdose
♦ The choice of drug must be tailored to each individual patient's circumstance
There is no general agreement about whether a tricyclic or a new antidepressant should be used first

Social – offer practical support and advice – e.g. refer to other agencies for advice on finances, housing etc

Reviewing the patient

♦ Acute treatment – review every 3–14 days as appropriate for individual
♦ Evaluate response – week 6
♦ If change in treatment – re-evaluate in 2 weeks
♦ Continuation treatment – see monthly for 6 months

Table 4.13 EHH health authority guidelines for management of depression in adults[18]

In order to prove their worth to clinicians, guidelines need to have a reliable evaluation tool to check them. Adjustments, if appropriate, can be made through this process. St George's Hospital Medical School has developed an appraisal instrument for clinical guidelines[20] to facilitate this process.

Before the implementation of locally agreed guidelines is initiated, other staff who have not been involved in the process need to be briefed on the final version. A start date made known to everyone needs to be agreed for the changes to come into effect.

The implementation of guidelines needs to be done by a number of people. An effective way of doing this is to devise an action plan which assigns responsibility for various actions to different types of staff. This way of supporting staff who are grappling with a new way of working is vital. A simple method of raising awareness is to encourage opinion leaders amongst staff to convey the message and ask for feedback on progress. Every opportunity should be taken to reinforce the message. The implementation should be a dynamic process, involving and listening to people and making notes on comments from those who are working with the guidelines. This aids the ownership and evaluation of the guidelines.

A formal method of evaluating guidelines is to audit them. Before initiating the change, a baseline audit should be undertaken to assess the clinical practice occurring before the guidelines were in place. This can be compared with the outcome after implementation. Periodic review of the guidelines should be done to reflect the practicalities of carrying out the guidelines, new evidence coming to light and feedback on audit results.

It is an expensive and time-consuming process to produce and implement clinical guidelines. Not only are many clinicians and managers taken away from their regular work (which must be covered) to initially attend a number of meetings to do this, but ensuring the implementation of the guidelines also requires training of other staff on the newly agreed methods of working as well as the audit process to monitor the use of the guidelines. It is important not to underestimate the time and effort needed to implement and evaluate the whole process.

Issues for consideration

Consider which guidelines are in place in your organisation (i.e. which conditions are covered).

- How have these guidelines been initiated?
- Who were the key players?
- How were others involved?

Appraisal of guidelines

The two main issues concerning the development of a good set of guidelines
are to reduce biases that may be inherent in their creation and to assess the
method of dissemination and implementation proposed.[21] Cluzeau and
colleagues[20] have produced and evaluated a generic appraisal instrument
which health professionals can use to assess the quality of guidelines.

The instrument addresses three major dimensions:

1. The rigour of development
   - Responsibility for guideline development
   - The composition of the guideline development group including the
     input of patients and carers
   - Identification and interpretation of evidence – the search strategy
     used to find the supporting evidence; ideally this should be a
     systematic review
   - Formulation of recommendations
   - Peer review
   - The process of updating
   - Overall assessment of the development process
2. Context and content
   - Objectives
   - Context – i.e. the target population
   - Clarity – presentation and clarity of the recommendations
   - Likely costs and benefits
3. Application
   - Guideline dissemination and implementation
   - Monitoring of guidelines/clinical audit.

The instrument has been refined further into the AGREE (Appraisal of
Guidelines Research and Evaluation in Europe) Instrument
(www.agreecollaboration.org). This has been developed by an international
group of researchers to assess the quality of guidelines in any disease area,
including diagnosis, health promotion, treatment or interventions. It is has
been designed to assess guidelines presented in paper or electronic format
and for use by the following groups:

- Policy makers – to help them decide which guidelines could be
  recommended for use in practice
- Guideline producers – the instrument provides a structured and rigorous
  development methodology and a self-assessment tool to ensure that
  guidelines are robust
- Health care providers – who wish to undertake their own assessment
  before adopting recommendations.

The criteria addressed include:

- Scope and purpose
- Stakeholder involvement
- Rigour of development
- Clarity and presentation
- Applicability
- Editorial independence
- Overall assessment.

Both full appraisal instruments are in the toolkit at the end of the book.

The Critical Appraisal Skills Programme also has checklists for critically appraising guidelines (available on www.sghms.ac.uk/phs/hceu/nhsguide.htm).

What makes a good set of guidelines?

The appraisal questions described above assess the process of development of guidelines. The next stage, however, is to decide how helpful those guidelines are.

Jackson and Feder[22] proposed three main components to look out for in assessing the usefulness of a clinical guideline:

1. The identification of key decisions and their consequences
2. A review of the relevant, valid evidence on the benefits, risks and costs of alternative decisions
3. The presentation of the evidence required to inform key decisions in a simple accessible format that is flexible to stakeholder preferences.

Developing these themes further, the *Effective Healthcare Bulletin* produced by the NHS Centre for Reviews and Dissemination[23] proposed that guidelines should aim to be:

- Valid – following the guidelines should lead to the expected results
- Reproducible – when using the same clinical evidence and methods of developing guidelines, another group should be able to come up with essentially similar recommendations
- Reliable – if given the same clinical circumstances, different health professionals should be able to interpret and apply the guidelines in the same manner
- Cost effective – following the recommendations should lead to improvements in health of patients at acceptable costs
- Representative – all the key stakeholders affected should be involved in the development of guidelines
- Clinical applicability – the patient populations defined in the guidelines

are targeted in accordance with scientific evidence or best clinical judgement

- Flexible – there should be identification and provision for any exceptions to the recommendations in the guidelines, and there should be an indication of how patient views and preferences are taken into account in the decision-making process
- Clear – the language used in the guidelines must be unambiguous, precise and understandable (definitions of terms should be included, if necessary)
- Meticulous and reviewable – there should be records of all the participants involved, the evidence and the methods used in the process of developing the guidelines; this should facilitate the later review of guidelines after a period of time, and the date for review should be identified at the time.

Issues for consideration

Consider the use of any guidelines in your organisation.

- Are they being used?
- If they are, what is it that has made them successful?
- If they are not, why not?

Cost effectiveness

Medical care is constantly changing and developing. New drugs and procedures or health technologies exert a constant pressure on health services. It is estimated that about 100 new prescription drugs are launched in the United Kingdom each year as well as new equipment and technologies, which are often implemented without an opportunity for proper evaluation as to their value or effectiveness. These new interventions are very expensive to develop; for example, currently a typical pharmaceutical company will invest about £200m to develop a new drug and bring it to the market. This process takes about 10-12 years as a number of hurdles have to be overcome (including clinical trials on human subjects) before a drug is deemed ready for the general health care market. It is not surprising, therefore, that ways of providing health care that involve the use of new drugs and procedures tend to be costly and when this is superimposed onto a situation where resources are finite, close examination of the merits of the new intervention must be made. The usual method of doing this is to compare the new drug or technology with the standard accepted practice, looking at the outcome of care for patients and the associated costs.

The Department of Health defines the cost effectiveness of a particular form of health care as depending upon the ratio of the costs of health care to its health outcome. Another way of looking at it is, how many people can I get better for the money I have available? This may not be such a simple question as it first appears. For example, for minimal access surgery, most of the economic evaluations that have been conducted so far suggest that it is that it is relatively expensive when compared to conventional surgery. The immediate conclusion would be that it is not a good buy for the NHS. The reasons for this are that the disposable equipment used is expensive, and the operation takes longer than conventional surgery. It also means that more surgeons and anaesthetists are needed to do the same number of operations. However, this means a reduction in bed occupancy. Nevertheless, keyhole surgery, from the patient's perspective, is a good buy because with this procedure the patient may only be off work for 2 weeks, as opposed to 6 weeks with a conventional operation. This has very important economic implications for the patient, particularly if they are self employed, and often for their employer.

Economic analysis

One of the main problems in dealing with the cost effectiveness of an intervention is that this type of literature is scarce, of variable quality, and may not be easy to interpret. Approaches to this problem range from double-blind multi-centre randomised control trials, to controlled trials without randomisation, to clinical opinion.

However, the picture is changing and, increasingly, in response to questions about the effective use of finite resources and which interventions provide the best value, economic analysis is a growing feature of clinical papers.

Economic analysis

- is a technique to aid decision making when choices have to be made due to the finite availability of resources
- helps in allocating resources, particularly when there are competing claims
- aims to maximise the benefit to society from the resources available.

There are four main methodologies used in economic analysis:

Cost minimisation

This method assumes that the effectiveness or outcomes of interventions are equal for a given condition and compares the direct costs of each intervention. This can be used, for example, in comparing the costs of two similar drugs which have, for a particular condition, an equal outcome.

Cost effectiveness

This method compares the costs and outcomes of alternative treatments within therapeutic categories (but not across categories). Outcomes are measured in units – such as number of cases identified, lives saved, complications avoided, symptom-free days – and are related to the direct costs of a procedure as a ratio; i.e. the cost per unit of effectiveness. This method can be used, for example, in comparing alternative options in buying treatments for conditions such as eating disorders and infertility treatment, and differs from cost minimisation in that it includes outcome measurement.

Cost utility

This method allows comparison between the relative efficiency of health care interventions for different conditions and uses mortality and morbidity data combined as a single measure. A typical example is the use of the Quality Adjusted Life Year (QALY) which is a measure of the quantity of life gained by treatment, adjusted by increases in the quality of life. This method can be used to compare different treatments such as hip operations, advice on smoking cessation and treatment for hypertension.

Cost benefit

This method determines the absolute benefit of various models of care and is considered to be the gold standard of economic analysis. All the benefits (direct, indirect and intangible) are valued in the same units as the costs of interventions or treatments – usually in monetary terms. This process provides information on whether the benefits of interventions outweigh their costs, and can be used for assessing different models of care (e.g. comparing the management of stroke patients in a general medical ward, a stroke unit and at home).

　　The National Institute for Clinical Excellence, as part of the assessment of new drugs and technologies, carries out an economic assessment of their impact on the NHS (see Chapter 1).

The next major step in the clinical effectiveness process is getting the evidence into practice, to ensure that the research findings are applied to patients in a routine clinical setting. The next chapter describes how this can be achieved.

References

1. Walshe K, Ham C 1997 Who's acting on the evidence? Health Service Journal 3 April: 22-25
2. Eldridge K, South N 1998 Slow-acting remedy. Health Service Journal 21 May: 24-25
3. Richardson R 1999 PA for the course? Health Service Journal 11 March: 26
4. Muir Gray J A 1998 Where's the chief knowledge officer? British Medical Journal 317: 832
5. Department of Health 1993 Improving clinical effectiveness [Executive letter: EL(93)115]. Department of Health, London
6. Department of Health 1996 Promoting clinical effectiveness: a framework for action in and through the NHS. Department of Health, London
7. The Royal College of Nursing 1996 Clinical effectiveness initiative: a strategic framework. Royal College of Nursing, London
8. Department of Health 1998 Research and development: towards an evidence base for health services, public health and social care. Department of Health, London
9. Culyer A 1994 Supporting research and development in the NHS. HMSO, London
10. NHS Executive 1997 R&D support funding for NHS providers for 1998/99, an invitation to bid. NHS Executive, London
11. The Secretary of State for Health 1998 Information for health. NHS Executive, London
12. Richardson W S, Wilson M C, Nishikawa J et al 1995 The well-built clinical question: a key to evidence-based decisions [editorial]. ACP J Club 123(3): A12-13
13. Gosfield A G 1995 Clinical practice guidelines and the law: applications and implications. Colloquium report on legal issues related to clinical practice guidelines. National Lawyers Association, Washington DC
14. Field M J, Lohr K N (eds) 1990 Clinical practice guidelines: directions for a new programme. National Academy Press, Washington DC
15. NHS Executive 1996 Clinical guidelines: using guidelines to improve patient care within the NHS. NHS Executive, London
16. Woolf S H, Grol R, Hutchinson A et al 1999 Potential benefits, limitations and harms of clinical guidelines. British Medical Journal 318: 527-530
17. Ealing, Hammersmith and Hounslow Health Authority Drug and Therapeutics Advisory Group 1995 Dyspepsia drugs. Ealing, Hammersmith and Hounslow

Health Authority, London

18. UK Alcohol Forum 2001 Guidelines for the management of alcohol problems in primary care and general psychiatry, 2nd edn. Tangent Medical Education, London

19. Ealing, Hammersmith and Hounslow Health Authority, Drug and Therapeutics Advisory Group 1997 Management of depression in adults. Ealing, Hammersmith and Hounslow Health Authority, London

20. Cluzeau F, Littlejohns P, Grimshaw J et al 1997 Appraisal instrument for clinical guidelines. St George's Hospital Medical School, London

21. Cluzeau F A, Littlejohns P, Grimshaw J M et al 1999 Development and application of a generic methodolgy to assess the quality of clinical guidelines. International Journal for Quality in Healthcare 11(1): 21-28

22. Jackson R, Feder G 1998 Guidelines for clinical guidelines: a simple, pragmatic strategy for guidelines development. British Medical Journal 317: 427-428

23. University of York, NHS Centre for Reviews and Dissemination 1994 Implementing clinical practice guidelines: can guidelines be used to improve clinical practice? Effective Healthcare Bulletin 1(8)

Critical Appraisal Skills Programme – Further reading

Gray J A M 1997 Evidence-based healthcare: how to make health policy and management decisions. Churchill Livingstone, Edinburgh

CASP and HCLU 1999 Evidence-based healthcare, a computer aided learning resource. Update Software, Oxford

CASP and HCLU 1999 Evidence-based healthcare, an open learning resource for healthcare professionals. Update Software, Oxford

Beaglehole R, Bonita R, Kjellstrom T 1993 Basic epidemiology. World Health Organisation, Geneva

5

Quality initiatives – the process of clinical effectiveness
Part two: getting the evidence into practice (evidence-based practice, care pathways and clinical audit)

Applying research evidence to clinical practice is not an easy process. Often the research evidence sits around for a number of years before it is taken up in routine practice, and the reasons for the slow response are multifaceted. Haynes and Haines[1] identified a number of barriers to the implementation of evidence-based medicine, including:

- the size and complexity of the research
- difficulties in developing evidence-based clinical policy
- difficulties in applying the evidence due to:
  - poor access to best evidence and guidelines
  - organisational barriers
  - poor continuing education programmes
  - poor compliance to treatments by patients.

The first two points were discussed in the last chapter, concerning equipping clinicians and managers with critical appraisal skills to assess the research evidence as well as taking note of systematic reviews that have been done by institutions such as the Cochrane Centre, and through the medium of well drawn-up guidelines. Access to the evidence is improving with the recognition for the need of a 'chief knowledge officer' to disseminate information to the rest of the organisation.

What is evidence-based medicine and evidence-based health care?

Evidence-based medicine is 'the process of systematically reviewing, appraising and using contemporaneous research findings as the basis for clinical decisions' (Rosenberg and Donald[2]).

Evidence-based health care aims to 'provide the means by which current best evidence from research can be judiciously and conscientiously applied in the prevention, detection and care of health disorders'.[3]

Apart from the barriers identified above, there are also changes in behaviour that are necessary to ensure the successful implementation of guidelines. A variety of interventions are required, leading to a behaviour change in those required to follow a different way of working.

Interventions to promote behavioural change among health professionals[4]

Consistently effective interventions:
- Educational outreach visits (for prescribing in North America)
- Reminders (manual or computerised)
- Multifaceted interventions (a combination that includes two or more of the following: audit and feedback, reminders, local consensus processes or marketing)
- Interactive educational meetings (participation of health care providers in workshops that include discussion or practice).

Interventions of variable effectiveness:
- Audit and feedback (or any summary of clinical performance)
- The use of local opinion leaders (practitioners identified by their colleagues as influential)
- Local consensus processes (inclusion of participating practitioners in discussions to ensure that they agree that the chosen clinical problem is important and the approach to managing the problem is appropriate)
- Patient mediated interventions (any intervention aimed at changing the performance of health care providers for which specific information was sought from or given to patients).

Interventions that have little or no effect:
- Educational materials (distribution of recommendations for clinical care, including clinical practice guidelines, audiovisual materials and electronic publications)
- Didactic educational meetings (such as lectures).

A change in behaviour can be reinforced by providing incentives to work in a different way. Incentives, such as financial reward, resource allocation, education and training, performance feedback and empowerment have been shown to be effective. As with the process of obtaining the commitment of stakeholders, incentives that are locally negotiated and agreed are more likely to succeed than those imposed from above (see Chapter 3).

Example

A PCG wants to promote effective prescribing amongst its constituent practices. It has 'top sliced' part of the overall prescribing budget for the PCG, and has used this to provide a local incentive scheme to encourage good practice. It has highlighted a couple of areas where improvements can be made and, incidentally, savings. For example, the PCG is promoting a change in the cimetidine to ranitidine prescribing ratio and encouraging more effective use of proton pump inhibitors for the management of peptic ulcer. The incentive is £1000 per GP if targets are met, which in a large practice of 10 GPs means that the money can be used to fund a nurse to do the assessments of patients.
(From Mid-Hampshire PCG)

Issues for consideration

- What interventions have been used in your organisation to achieve a change in practice?

An example of evidence-based practice

In Bradford, the chief dietician (Loach, personal communication), who had studied the application of evidence-based practice, decided to set up a similar process for her dietetic colleagues in the area. When the idea was first aired with the local dieticians, the reactions included concerns over the lack of skills, time and resources for individuals to pursue the process, and a questioning of the purpose of evidence-based practice. The solution was to encourage the discussion of the process in a group format so that the work was shared amongst a number of clinicians. This was initiated by a workshop for all dieticians in the locality, which covered the principles and rationale of evidence-based practice. From that session, a smaller group was identified to take the next steps, using the following questions as a guide:

- What questions do we want answers to?
- Where do we find the evidence?
- Who will do what, by when?
- Which topics could be used for an initial study?

A large number of topics were initially identified for study, from which a small number were identified for further examination. The topics were either 'grey' areas of dietetics – not necessarily the main workload, but the cause of persistent referrals in the belief that dietary modification had a role – or areas where, as a department, there were no specialist practitioners.

Topics identified by Bradford dieticians for evidence-based study

- Irritable bowel syndrome
- Crohn's disease
- Arthritis
- Migraine
- Gout
- Attention-deficit hyperactivity disorder
- Cholecystitis – is a low fat diet of benefit?
- Acid reflux – are any dietary measures of benefit?
- Renal stones
- Wound care
- Calcium – can calcium supplements be used to treat osteoporosis?
- Hypertension – can a reduced sodium intake reduce blood pressure in an individual?
- Effectiveness of healthy eating interventions
- Vitamin E supplements and diabetes.

The main criterion for selection was those areas that had been agreed as local priorities. The diagram below illustrates the different points in the process of evidence-based practice that were developed by the dieticians, and the role of the group in implementing the key tasks.

The main benefit of working as a group was that no one was operating in isolation; ideas were generated and support provided from different members. It also provided an opportunity for discussion of the available evidence and a comparison of different methods of disseminating clinically relevant research.

One of the main obstacles faced by the dieticians was that very little of the research evidence was relevant to dietetics, making selection of the evidence difficult. Any evidence that existed was focused mostly on the work of doctors and nurses. This conclusion was reached after the group sifted through a vast quantity of information. There was a danger that interpretation of the evidence was prone to be subjective or biased, and this raised more questions than answers. Overall, it was time consuming.

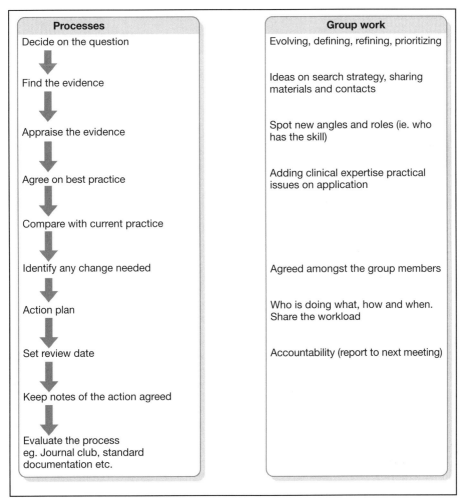

Processes	Group work
Decide on the question	Evolving, defining, refining, prioritizing
Find the evidence	Ideas on search strategy, sharing materials and contacts
Appraise the evidence	Spot new angles and roles (ie. who has the skill)
Agree on best practice	Adding clinical expertise practical issues on application
Compare with current practice	
Identify any change needed	Agreed amongst the group members
Action plan	Who is doing what, how and when. Share the workload
Set review date	Accountability (report to next meeting)
Keep notes of the action agreed	
Evaluate the process eg. Journal club, standard documentation etc.	

Figure 5.1 Flow chart illustrating different points in the process of evidence-based practice that were developed by dieticians, and the role of the group in implementing key tasks

However, the project did stimulate much interest and activity, including encouraging the following:

- Baseline audits of current practice
- Resource developments and updates (e.g. journal club)
- Dissemination of information activity to the public, referrers and other health professionals
- Further questions
- The development of guidelines, including referral criteria and treatment protocols and standard documentation

- Input to multi-professional/multi-agency guidelines (e.g. hypertension and wound care)
- Informed future training and education programmes.

Evaluation of the workshops revealed that although there were various pros and cons, the overall outcome was that the dieticians considered this an important process to help them improve patient care.

Table 5.1 Evaluation of the evidence-based process as experienced by Bradford dieticians	
What is good about the process?	**What is difficult about the process?**
Ensures practice moves forward	Vast amount of information – need to be selective and to summarise succinctly
Useful update on unfamiliar topics	Open to be subjective/biased
Informs policy updates and training	Very little information
Highlights the importance of evidence-based practice	Often left with more questions than answers
Shows the strengths and weaknesses of current practice	Cannot/does not always answer the specific questions set
Gives credibility and confidence	Time consuming
Gained experience of electronic databases	
Learnt a process of collecting information and how to arrive at a conclusion	
Saves time	

Although this example of evidence-based practice considers dieticians, the principles of the process and outcomes are applicable to other health professionals.

Issues for consideration

- Are you aware of any activity in your organisation that has/is addressing evidence-based practice?
- What are the key factors in the success of the initiative?

Care pathways – a method for implementing evidence-based practice

Implementing evidence-based practice, even if it is via the medium of guidelines and incentives, is a difficult process, particularly if a number of different disciplines, each with their own traditions, training and background, are required to work together in a manner with which they are unfamiliar. The main problem is that of communication – between the different professionals in a team (e.g. doctor, nurse, physiotherapist etc.); between members of the same profession (e.g. consultant and junior doctor or sister and staff nurse); between different departments in the same trust (e.g. accident and emergency and admitting wards); across health care sectors (such as primary and secondary care and mental health); and general communication between health services, social services and the voluntary sector – while providing 'seamless' care for patients.

The main fear in implementing guidelines is the generation of yet more paperwork, interfering with patient care and increasing the risk of litigation. The latter is dealt with in more detail in Chapter 6.

As clinical care becomes more complex, it is imperative to have a systematic way of controlling the processes of how that health care is delivered. This process needs to be flexible enough to be modified as new evidence comes to light, to be examined for critical review and to be amenable to audit. One tool that is increasingly being used to tackle this problem is the use of care pathways. In 1999, around 250 organisations in the NHS and independent sector were piloting the use of pathways or were fully implementing them in all kinds of medical, surgical and mental health specialties. Pathways are also being developed in the general practice setting.

What are care pathways?

The concept came originally from Boston's New England Medical Centre in the USA in 1983. Four core questions were posed by the project team:

- What is required by each profession to bring patients with similar diagnoses to realistic outcomes?
- What is the best way to produce that work?
- Who is accountable for those outcomes?
- How can we restructure care so that this happens in a consistent manner?

The outcome of the project was a one-page tool that detailed clinical interventions and a timeline called a critical path or Caremap®. These were to be used to chart more precisely the care patients receive in hospital, and for assessing the clinical and cost effectiveness of various specific treatments or procedures. The concept was introduced in the United Kingdom in 1989 as part of a resource management initiative undertaken by North West Thames Regional Health Authority. It was then adapted and developed for the NHS setting. Various names have been ascribed to the tool; for example, multidisciplinary pathways of care, protocols, integrated care pathways, critical care paths, anticipated recovery pathways and pathways of care. Generally, the term 'care pathways' is used nowadays.

Definition of a care pathway[5]

An integrated care pathway determines locally agreed, multidisciplinary practice based on guidelines and evidence where available, for a specific patient/client group. It forms all or part of the clinical record, documents the care given and facilitates the evaluation of outcomes for continuous quality improvement.

The essential feature of care pathways is that the process is built from current clinical practice, including any guidelines that are available, and is produced by the professional team that is involved in the care of the specific patient group identified. It reflects actual practice as discussed and agreed by the team involved, and charts the interventions made by different health professionals for any period of time in the care of specific patients. The process used in the development and refinement of care pathways is illustrated below. Note that this is similar to the audit and 'do and review' cycle.

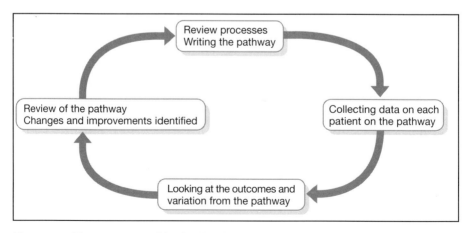

Figure 5.2 The process used in the development and refinement of care pathways

Aims of care pathways[6]

The aims of care pathways are to:
- facilitate the introduction of guidelines and systematic, dynamic audit into clinical practice
- improve multidisciplinary communication and planning of care
- reach or exceed existing quality standards
- reduce unwanted variation in clinical practice
- improve communication between clinicians and patients
- improve patient satisfaction
- identify research and development questions.

How are pathways developed?

The following steps describe the process of putting together a pathway.

1. Select an important area of practice. The topic area could include common or costly conditions, conditions where there is a high level of interest amongst local staff, and conditions where variations in practice occur that affect patient outcomes. These may have been identified in the clinical governance action plan for the organisation. In addition, selection could be from the priorities identified nationally (e.g. the National Service Frameworks, Our Healthier Nation or the Health Improvement Programme).

2. Gather support for the project. This is vital for the pathway to work effectively. Using the process of identification of the relevant stakeholders (see Chapter 3) will enhance the chance of success of the project.

3. Review practice. An exercise in reviewing current practice, for example through audit and any other relevant information such as guidelines, will provide the basis for interprofessional discussions.

4. Define the team. This is the identification of the multidisciplinary team who will be involved in providing the care for the condition selected. The team will also be responsible for developing and implementing the pathway based on actual practice achievable locally.

5. Define the case type/client group. Within the topic area selected, there needs to be an agreement on the exact patient condition for which a pathway is to be developed. For example, for a myocardial infarction, the case type could be management in the community, with the emergency services, within the accident and emergency department (A&E), in the coronary care unit (CCU) or for cardiac rehabilitation. For surgical pathways, the case type could be for a single procedure such as

a total hip replacement or for a group of similar conditions which have essentially the same interventions (e.g. minor and major gynaecological surgery). It is always better to start with a small, well-defined case type or client group in order to enhance the likelihood of success.

6. Agree the time frame. The time frame defines the points at which the pathway begins and ends; for example, an A&E pathway would be from admission to A&E to admission to the admitting ward (i.e. a matter of hours). Similarly, a pathway in the ward would be from admission to discharge, although the time frame would be a period of days. For pathways in the community setting the time frame can be up to a year, reflecting the chronic nature of some conditions (e.g. diabetes).

7. Agree the goals/outcomes of care. There could be a number of outcomes, depending on the opinion and experience of the team. These can be categorised into clinical, managerial or administrative outcomes: for example, ensuring that every patient is started on thrombolytic therapy within half an hour of admission in A&E; or looking at the use of resources (are there unnecessary treatments or duplication of effort by different clinical staff?); or is there enough of the right equipment at the right time available to treat patients with an acute abdominal pain? It is advisable to keep the number of outcomes low to assess the effect of the pathway on the condition studied.

8. Drawing up the pathway. Once the team has decided the above criteria, the pathway can then be written. The method is to identify, in a systematic manner, the tasks each member of the team has to perform for a patient presenting with the condition, through the above process and within the time scales decided. The key, here, is to document what is actually done and also the standards the team members have identified. Guidelines or looking at the research evidence can help here if people are not sure. The aim is to draw up a grid on one sheet of paper summarising the interventions that should be carried out in the time frame agreed upon by the team. Examples of pathways are illustrated in Tables 5.2, 5.3 and 5.4.

9. Training. Before the pathway can 'go live', all the staff who will be using the pathway need to be informed of the appropriate use of the tool.

10. Piloting the pathway. Testing the pathway on a small number of patients or for a short period of time (e.g. 3 or 6 months) will iron out discrepancies and ensure that staff are confident in using the tool.

11. Implementing the pathway. Once the above steps have been carried out, implementation can begin. A careful check needs to be made to assess the level of recording of information on the pathway.

Table 5.2 Integrated care pathway for diabetes[7]

Name: ....

Address: ....   G.P.:

D.O.B.: ....   Date of diagnosis: ....

PLEASE DATE AND SIGN THE BOXES

Day 1 (Visit 1)	1 week (Visit 2)	2 weeks-1 month (Visit 3)	3 months (Visit 4)	6 months (Visit 5)	1 year (Visit 6)
General Practitioner Confirm diagnosis (BMSTIX > 10mmol/L) Send investigations Preliminary educational material. Start treatment. ☐	Inform patient of diagnosis. Implications to life style. ☐	Review appointment ☐	Review appointment ☐	Review appt. ☐	**ANNUAL REVIEW** ☐
Practice Nurse Health check. Urine result. Initial basic education and advice. ☐	Referral to: Diabetes Nurse Specialist Dietitian Chiropodist Optometrist Refer to BDA **Give patient held card.** ☐	Review appointment ☐	Review appt. ☐	Review appt. ☐	**ANNUAL REVIEW** ☐
Receptionist Ensure notes available. Registration forms. Urine bottle Temporary tag. Diabetic register. ☐	Phone for results. Temporary tag to permanent tag. ☐				
Diabetic Nurse Specialist	Patient to attend for hospital education session ☐				Appt. as necessary ☐
Dietitian		Assess patient. Treatment if appropriate. Follow up if necessary. ☐			Annual assessment ☐
Chiropodist		Assess patient. Treatment if appropriate. Follow up if necessary. ☐			Annual assessment ☐
Optometrist	Can be seen straight away. ☐				Annual assessment ☐
Patient	To inform the practice of a named **Pharmacist**				

Table 5.3 Acute exacerbation of COPD care pathway (day 2) (Central Middlesex Hospital)

Patient name	DAY 2 = Day:	Date:	Ward

Contact Thoracic team or ITU Reg/SHO if evidence of decompensated respiratory failure

MILESTONES/OUTCOMES MET If no please give reason
- ■ Able to speak sentences ☐
- ■ Mobile bed to chair ☐

ASSESSMENT		Better	Same	Worse
■ Conscious level		☐	☐	☐
■ Able to speak sentences		☐	☐	☐
■ Purulent sputum *(If YES confirm culture sent)*		☐	☐	☐
■ Peripheral oedema		☐	☐	☐

- ■ VAS score completed. <u>Please use separate sheet for each day.</u>   Yes ☐   No ☐

- ■ Monitor·   Vital signs; fluid balance; daily weight ____ kg
  Peak flow pre and post nebuliser
  Pulse oximetry (state O_2 concentration ____ %)

- ■ **Waterlow:**   **< 10** ☐   Other _____
  If at risk: Relieve pressure ____ hrly *(Describe pressure points opposite)*
  Equipment:

INVESTIGATIONS	Yes	No	Comments:
■ U + Es if abnormal on Day 1	☐	☐	
■ ABG: *Repeat if Type II*	☐	☐	

DRUGS
- ■ Administer nebulisers
- ■ Review steroid therapy 24 hrs after admission
  (Continue Prednisolone if documented evidence of reversibility or new patient)

MANAGEMENT		Yes	No
■ **Care plan** discussed and explained to patient by: _____ (sign)			
■ **Inhaler:** Drug: Device: Component		☐	☐
■ **Seen by physiotherapist**		☐	☐
■ **Refer to CCT for early discharge assessment**		☐	☐
■ If accepted by CCT, arrange OPA for 4/52		☐	☐
■ **Discharge:** does patient meet social criteria for discharge:		☐	☐

  (Independent ADLs/Able to climb stairs/Able to self medicate/Has sufficient home support)
  If no refer to   OT ☐   Social Services ☐

- ■ **ADLs:** *Please indicate – Independent/Equipment req./Assistance req./Not assessed*
  Transfers: Bed ____ Chair ____ Toilet ____ Bath ____
  Selfcare: Washing ____ Dressing ____ Toileting ____ Feeding ____
  Exercise Tolerance: _____

RGN: AM	PM	NIGHT

©1995 Central Middlesex NHS Trust (THOR/COPD/003/1198/VM/CC)

PRE-MORBID BASELINE

Mental state:

Mobility:

Transfers: Bed _____ Chair _____ Toilet _____ Bath _____

Selfcare: Washing _____ Dressing _____ Toileting _____ Feeding _____

Please indicate – Independent/Equipment req./Assistance req./Not assessed

Shoppping:

Cooking/cleaning:

| RGN: AM | PM | NIGHT |

Date + Time	MULTIDISCIPLINARY PROGRESS NOTES	Signature + Profession

Date + Time	VARIANCE	REASON FOR VARIATION	ACTION	Signature + Profession

Table 5.4 Gynaecology surgery care pathway

POST-OP DAY 2 Date:		NAME: _____ HOSPITAL NUMBER: _____
MILESTONES:		**REASONS IF NOT MET @ 4pm:**
■ Apyrexial	Y/N	
■ Hb >10.5g/dl and no clinical symptoms of anaemia	Y/N	
■ Passing urine normally	Y/N	
■ Bowels open	Y/N	
■ Evidence of wound healing	Y/N	
■ Pain-free with or without analgesia	Y/N	
■ Independently mobile	Y/N	
ASSESSMENT		
■ Vital signs; Fluid balance; Pain; Bowels		
INVESTIGATIONS		
■ FBC Y/N Result:		
■ Remove venflon (If blood transfusion not required). Removed	Y/N	
■ Is patient pyrexial? (2–3° rise above baseline recorded pre-surgery)	Y/N	
If YES		
Review blood count, wound and chest.		
Consider blood cultures (Ideally 3 separate samples NOT taken through the IV line)	Y/N	
Consider urine sample (Infection unlikely to be caused by a catheter if only in situ	Y/N	
for 24 hours especially if the patient has received prophylactic antibiotics)		
DRUGS		
■ Obtain TTQs		
■ Sodium heparin 5000 iu sc twice daily	Y/N	
■ If additional antibiotics are required the PR route for Flagyl is recommended		
until oral doses are tolerated		
MANAGEMENT		
■ Walk to washroom to carry out ADLs	Y/N	
■ Check TEDs used correctly and heels not discoloured	Y/N	
■ Normal diet	Y/N	
■ Wound: Abdominal: Dressing checked and satisfactory	Y/N	
Vaginal: Check PV loss not excessive	Y/N	
■ Confirm patient for CCT + commence discharge checklist		
AM PM NT		

© Copyright Central Middlesex Hospital NHS Trust (Gynaecology/Major Surgery/06/0898/HW; NG)

Pathways have developed in a number of ways since their introduction to the NHS. For example, some pathways contain a space for the patient's input to their own care (usually relating to whether they understand the treatment they are receiving) and some have incorporated into the pathway the consent form for the patient to agree to the care proposed.

The Central Middlesex Hospital has developed the tool to such a degree that the pathway has become part of the patient's notes, and is used by all the health professionals involved in that care.

Table 5.5 Examples of pathways in use in a hospital setting (Central Middlesex Hospital, London)[8]

Medicine	Surgery	Accident and Emergency
Asthma	Fractured neck of femur	Postcoital contraception
Cardiac chest pain	Total joint replacements – hips and knees	Nasal injury and epistaxis
Acute sickle cell crisis	Transurethral resection of the prostate	Ankle injury
Diabetic ketoacidosis	Hysterectomy – vaginal and abdominal	
Chronic obstructive pulmonary disease	Miscarriage or ectopic pregnancy < 18 weeks	
Stroke	Ear, nose and throat – short stay pathway – includes grommets, submucosal diathermy, tonsillectomy, myringotomy, bilateral atrium washout, adenotonsillectomy, dewaxing, examination under anaesthetic postnasal space	

Setting up a system for noting the variations from the pathway

Patients react differently to the treatments they receive for their conditions. The pathway that will have been drawn up will chart the expected course in the majority of patients. However, situations may occur that do not follow the pathway. This is to be expected, and can be classified as avoidable,

unavoidable or a combination of both. Avoidable variations from the
pathway could, for example, include a delay in getting a prescription ready
in time for discharge, which may necessitate a further day's stay in hospital
because the hospital pharmacy has closed, or unavoidable variations such
as further clinical complications (e.g. the development of a post-operative
infection). Noting these variations in the expected clinical care is an
important aspect of the pathway and forms the basis of clinical audit.

Reasons for variation from the pathway[6]

- Patient's clinical condition
- Patient's social circumstances
- Associated conditions
- Changing technology or techniques
- Clinician's decision not to follow the pathway
- Internal system: services or consultations from other departments within the organisation
- External system: services or consultations from social services or other health care sectors.

Patient name				Variation tracking sheet		
Date	Day no	Time	Variation and reason for it	Variation code	Action taken	Signature
1. Patient condition 2. Patient's family & carers 3. Staff/people 4. System 5. Other						

Table 5.6 Example of a variation sheet

Each pathway will have a variation sheet attached to it. Pathways that have
developed further have a space for variations to be noted as part of the
pathway itself (see, for example, the pathways from Central Middlesex
Hospital illustrated above).

In the hospital setting, the pathway is usually placed at the end of the patient's bed so that everybody (including the patient) knows what is happening and what should happen next. The member of staff responsible for a particular intervention demonstrates that they have done this by signing against the procedure on the pathway; for example, the nurses who give the medication should sign their name against that part of the pathway. Anything that does not follow the pathway is noted on the variation sheet and the source of it is identified, referring to the code numbers at the bottom of the variation sheet. For example, a urinary catheter may not have been removed from a patient on the day of discharge when it should have been out earlier; this would be classified under staff (or code 3 in this case) as this was a staff responsibility. Alternatively, the patient may have some blood test results which are taking longer than expected to return to normal levels; this would be noted under patient condition (or code 1); in this case the patient would come off the pathway and be treated as appropriate.

An assessment of the frequency of variation from the pathways that occur will provide a guide to the main issues that need to be addressed. The variations can be presented graphically for feedback to the team. This is the review part of the audit cycle, and it provides an opportunity to check that the standards or outcomes that have been set are appropriate. Any conclusions arising from the discussion can then be incorporated into the pathway when it is next reviewed. For the pathway to have the greatest impact, regular reviews of the variations that occur should be discussed amongst the team members.

In the community setting, patient-held cards can be used as the pathway. There are examples of patient-held cards already in existence (e.g. the cards held by pregnant mothers holding the information on their antenatal care, and the parent-held records for children under five years of age). The cards are useful in that the patient can take their record with them and present it to any health professional looking after them wherever they are located in the community.

Patient-held cards encourage the patients themselves to take an interest in their condition. The simple layout of the cards shows patients what to expect during their treatments and when it should happen. The cards encourage patients and their carers to ask questions about the rationale for their particular medications or investigations. Patients who understand their condition and are involved in decision making concerning their treatment are more likely to be motivated to take care of themselves – i.e. a change in emphasis to patients taking responsibility for their own health.

There is a national organisation, called the National Pathways

Association, whose members have developed care pathways in a number of settings and are using the tool to improve the quality of clinical care provided and to support the development of clinical governance. Further details can be found on their website (http://www.the-npa.org.uk).

Effectiveness of pathways

There is much research on benefits, concerns and barriers to care pathways.[6]

Table 5.7 Benefits, concerns and barriers of care pathways[7]

Benefits

- Facilitates the application of the research evidence into practice
- Better and accessible data collection for audit, and encourages change in practice
- Promotes multidisciplinary communication and care planning – reducing the duplication of effort
- Promotes patient-centred care and patient information and improves record keeping
- Reduces the size of the case notes
- Enables new staff to learn rapidly the key interventions for specific conditions and to be aware of likely variations
- Promotes multidisciplinary audit and prompt incorporation of improvements in care into routine practice

Concerns

- Time consuming in the initial stages
- May discourage clinical judgement in individual cases
- Difficult to develop in circumstances where there are multiple pathologies or where clinical management is very variable
- May stifle innovation/ progress if poorly applied
- Need leadership, enthusiasm and good communication and time for successful implementation
- May be misused – e.g. management may interpret the pathway in such a way as to reduce patient care costs inappropriately

Barriers

- Reluctance to change
- Lack of suitable existing evidence-based guidelines, inadequate time and resources for local development
- Obstructive interpersonal politics
- The person responsible for co-ordinating the setting up of the pathways must be well informed about the process and of a high enough standing within the organisation

Layton and colleagues[8] were able to demonstrate a number of changes following the introduction of pathways in their hospital. These included achieving various clinical milestones set for the conditions and reduction in lengths of stay. These achievements were attributed to the setting up of a collaborative care team, which resulted in the improved co-ordination of care and the provision of continued support for patients at home. The average length of stay for many groups of patients fell by up to 4 days. For example, over a course of 2 years, the average stay for a patient having a total knee replacement fell from 12 to 7 days, and for an abdominal hysterectomy from 6 to 3 days.

Table 5.8 Examples of milestones met using pathways[4]

Milestone targets met	1995 (%)	1996 (%)	1997 (%)
Post-myocardial infarction			
Aspirin on discharge*	98	99	99
β blockers on discharge*	93	95	95
Cardiac rehabilitation*	83	95	96
Acute sickle cell crisis			
Intramuscular analgesia within			
15 minutes of arrival at A&E	10	67	63
Primigravida mothers receiving anti-D			
28 weeks		65**	96
36 weeks		77**	100
Post-natal		69**	100
Abdominal hysterectomy			
Operated on day of admission	3	83	94
Miscarriage			
Operated on within 24 hours of			
confirmation of miscarriage	40	96	89

*   pathway implemented in 1993; limited data available pre-pathway
** before implementation of pathway.

De Luc (personal communication) conducted a formal before and after study of the effectiveness of two care pathways at the Kidderminster Healthcare NHS Trust. One pathway focused on the diagnosis following the discovery of a breast lump, from GP referral to continued surgical treatment, or discharge if no intervention was required; the other focused on midwifery-led care of multigravida mothers from the first antenatal booking to the hand-over to the health visitor (usually 10 days post-natally). The outcomes of clinical care are shown in Table 5.9.

Table 5.9 The effectiveness of two care pathways at Kidderminster Healthcare NHS Trust

Breast disease clinical care			Midwifery-led maternity clinical care		
	Control	Pathway		Control	Pathway
Percentage of patients having two to three OPD visits for diagnosis	26	13*	Reduced number of GP antenatal contacts (mean)	5.1	3.8*
Waiting time for diagnostic surgery (mean number of days)	16.5	9.8	Increased number of midwifery antenatal contacts (mean)	8.1	9.1*
Percentage of cancer patients first seeing SBCN	13	61	Length of stay (days)	2.2	2.1**
Establishment of multidisciplinary meetings (%)	0	72	Reduced number of midwifery post-natal contacts (mean)	9.0	8.7**
Number of days to report mammogram result to patient (mean number of days)	7.1	1.7*	Percentage of mothers having 10 visits	40	30
Waiting time to be seen in OPD (mean number of days)	10.3	10.2**	Increased percentage of women breast feeding	55	64**
Waiting times for therapeutic surgery (mean number of days)	8.3	8.8**			
Number of times SBCN saw cancer patients (mean)	2.3	2.2**			

*statistically significant; **not statistically significant; SBCN, specialist breast care nurse.

The results of the study were mixed, both in terms of clinical care and of patient and staff satisfaction with the process. The momentum for the change in care was greatest at the beginning of the project, highlighting a need for the continuous commitment of time and effort required to maintain the operation of the pathways. This should be facilitated by the direction and support provided by the clinical governance agenda.

Issues for consideration

- Are pathways used in your organisation? If so, for what purpose?
- How can pathways be used as a means for implementing the process of clinical governance in your organisation?

A specific database and research literature on pathways has been set up and can be accessed through the National Electronic Library for Health www.nelh.nhs.uk.

Clinical audit

Many health professionals recognise the need to perform clinical audit to check that what they think they are doing is what is actually happening. Audit is a means of measuring the care that is being provided in day-to-day clinical practice. The process provides an objective method of doing this, as perceptions do not necessarily reflect real life. Audit will also show whether the research findings can actually be applied in practice; for example, many randomised controlled trials exclude female patients. There are other exclusions, such as age or other concurrent pathologies or aspects of the social situation, which narrows the field even more.

The NHS reforms in 1989[9] highlighted the need for audit in clinical practice supported by earmarked funding. Initially this focused almost exclusively on the work of doctors, but the policy was soon revised to include nurses and professions allied to medicine,[10] and the concept of multidisciplinary audit was introduced.

> Clinical audit has been defined by the Department of Health as 'the systematic and critical analysis of the quality of clinical care, including the procedures for the diagnosis, treatment and care, the associated use of resources and the resulting outcome and quality of life for the patient'.[11]

The process of clinical audit is best illustrated as an audit cycle. This forms a building block of clinical governance. The essence of audit is to examine the data that has been collected concerning a defined standard, usually from patients' notes, in order to measure the actual clinical care given. If the audit reveals that the defined standard has been achieved, then the process can be applied to another area of practice. It is important to remember that an audit is a snapshot in time, and that for an assessment of improvement in care a dynamic process is necessary.

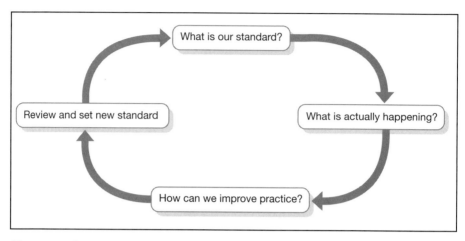

Figure 5.3 Process of clinical audit

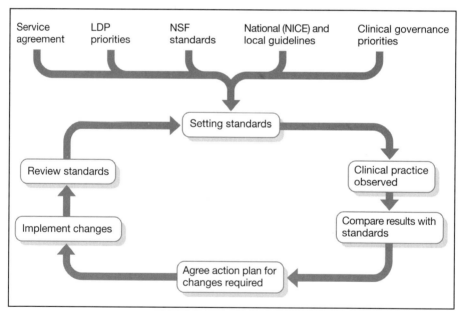

Figure 5.4 Audit cycle in the context of national policies

An example of an audit process[12]

The Berkshire Audit Group held a county-wide workshop for all disciplines in the primary and secondary care setting who worked with stroke and transient ischaemic attack patients. The topic was chosen as it is identified as a priority in the government's White Paper *Saving Lives: Our Healthier*

Nation. In primary care the agreement was to look at the prevention of strokes by treating hypertensive patients effectively and patients with atrial fibrillation with either anticoagulation or aspirin. The audits and expected standards are shown in Table 5.10.

Audit one – hypertension	Audit two – atrial fibrillation
Aim: To identify all hypertensives between 60 and 80 years of age and to control their hypertension adequately in order to reduce the incidence of stroke in Berkshire	Aim: To reduce the incidence of stroke in Berkshire by treating patients with atrial fibrillation with aspirin or anticoagulation
Criterion 1: All patients aged between 40 and 80 years should have a recorded blood pressure reading within the last 3 years Standard: 80%	Criterion 1: All patients with atrial fibrillation should be identified Standard: 80%
Criterion 2: All hypertensives aged between 60 and 80 years should be identified (i.e. known patients with hypertension and/or a blood pressure reading greater than 140/90) Standard: 90%	Criterion 2: All patients with atrial fibrillation are either on aspirin or anticoagulation unless contraindicated Standard: 90%
Criterion 3: All hypertensives (i.e. known patients with hypertension and/or a blood pressure reading greater than 140/90) aged between 60 and 80 years should be controlled with a blood pressure of 160/90 or below Standard: 50%	

Table 5.10 Audits and expected standards from *Saving Lives: Our Healthier Nation*

The following information on how to conduct the audits was provided to (the then) PCGs in the Berkshire area:

1. Identify the audit team
2. Identify the patient population aged 40-80 years (male and female)
3. Run a computer search to identify the blood pressure readings or undertake a manual search
4. Complete the data forms provided and send back the summary findings to the Medical Audit Advisory Group
5. A report is produced once the analysis has been completed (the data remains confidential).

Support to the process of clinical audit was provided by the Berkshire Medical Audit Advisory Group in terms of funding and analysis of the information. The information was fed back to the individual practices for discussion of the findings, and for the local PCGs to determine the appropriate action plan to improve clinical care.

Some clinical audit outcomes – examples[11]

- An audit of asthma management in primary care showed that the introduction of a nurse-run asthma clinic led to a 42% increase in routine asthma checks, a 236% increase in the use of prophylactic medication and a resultant 209% increase in peak flow measurements. In another audit, the improvements that occurred included a 67% reduction in the number of days lost from work by patients with asthma and a 68% reduction in acute attacks.
- After one audit into the management of a gastrointestinal bleed, a shared care protocol between primary and secondary care was introduced. Mortality reduced from 13% to 4%.
- In one Accident and Emergency department, X-rays of nasal fractures are no longer routinely taken when an audit showed that they did not influence subsequent treatment.
- An audit of the effectiveness of a multidisciplinary pain relief service in a hospital led to the appointment of a clinical nurse specialist and subsequent improvement of 20% in the management of pain.

Barriers to getting involved in clinical audit include:[13]

- hierarchical nurse-doctor relationships
- poor organisational links or conflicts between departments of quality and departments of audit in acute and community providers
- lack of commitment from senior nurses or managers in supporting nursing audit
- workload pressures and lack of protected time
- poor delegation of the workload
- availability or lack of uptake of practical support
- lack of knowledge and skills to undertake effective audit
- competing priorities for continuing education; audit training a low priority.

The value of audit has been recognised within the NHS, with specific funding for the process. There is also a contractual obligation for health professionals to participate in clinical audit. (NB: Currently GPs are not required to do so; however, it is considered good practice to participate, and many do.)

For many organisations and individuals, the main barriers to getting involved in clinical audit, as with other quality improvement processes, are time and resources. It is in this area that incentives for encouraging health professionals are well developed.

Incentives for clinical audit – example

A PCG is funding specific audit activity in line with the recommendations of the National Service Framework for coronary heart disease. Practices are given some money up front to do systematic case finding on patients who need to be on aspirin or beta-blocker treatment for various coronary heart disease conditions. Once the audit has been completed, practices are then eligible for the remainder of their allocated funding.
(From Mid-Hampshire PCG)

Planning and designing a clinical audit

Setting up a clinical audit requires careful planning, and needs to involve a number of elements. The National Centre for Clinical Audit, part of the National Institute for Clinical Excellence, provides guidance on good practice in clinical audit for clinicians intending to carry out clinical audits, for local or national audit groups or committees, or for purchasers funding audit programmes.

The Centre has produced a checklist to help in the planning of an audit in order that each of the five steps in the process is systematically followed[14] (the full checklist is in the toolkit at the end of the book). Note that planning and designing a clinical audit is not unlike the change management process.

Design

- Involve stakeholders – it is important that stakeholders in a service have the opportunity to contribute ideas for audits and that they are involved in the audit process as appropriate
- Select an important topic – the topics selected should relate to an important aspect of the quality of care and to national priorities (e.g. the Health Improvement Programme, NHS Plan priorities, National Service Framework standards etc.)
- State objectives – the objectives should be small in number (one or two) and they should be defined clearly and focused
- Use explicit measures – these enable comparison between the actual practice currently happening and the good practice desired

- Reflect good practice – the audit objectives and measures should reflect the best available evidence of good practice
- Define case selection – the number, type of cases and the time period over which the audit is to cover should be clear.

Measure

- Test validity and reliability of data – the data to be collected should be valid and reliable to enable a comparison between current and good practice
- Respect ethics and confidentiality – ethical principles must be followed and there should be regard for confidentiality of patient information
- Analyse audit data – the analysis should provide a complete, unbiased and accurate picture of actual practice.

Evaluate

- Present audit data – presentation of the results should be clear and easily understood
- Identify shortcomings and their causes – this is the identification of problems in the provision of clinical care, comparing actual practice and good practice
- Identify needed improvements – these should be related to the audit objectives and in line with recognised good practice.

Act

- Devise a strategy for action – this is the action plan for implementing the identified improvements in practice
- Implement action – the successful implementation of the action plan should be assessed (e.g. from feedback from the stakeholders).

Repeat for improvement

- Repeat the process – this is the repeat of the above processes until the desired level of quality has been achieved and sustained.

Part of the feedback of the clinical audit process is the production of a clinical audit report to demonstrate the activities that have taken place over the past year and to show the resultant improvements in the quality of clinical care. This is an important component of the clinical governance report. The London Regional Office of the NHS Executive has developed one such report, which is outlined below (the full template is in the toolkit at the end of the book).

Draft template of clinical audit report for a trust board[15]

The clinical audit programme:

- background
- selection of topics
- monitoring the programme
- costs
- critical analysis
- recommendations for action.

The individual audits, it is suggested, should be attached as annexes to the clinical audit report and should contain the following information:

- title
- participants
- standards
- objectives
- methods
- findings
- action
- costs follow-up
- recommendations.

Apart from the National Centre for Clinical Audit, there other organisations that support clinical audit on a national level, including:[16]

- The Clinical Resource and Audit Group (CRAG) in Edinburgh
- The Eli Lilly National Clinical Audit Centre in Leicester
- The Medical and Surgical Royal Colleges
- The Royal College of Nursing
- The British Psychological Society
- The Chartered Society of Physiotherapy
- The College of Occupational Therapists
- The Community Practitioners' and Health Visitors' Association
- The Faculty of Dental Surgery
- The Medical Research Council
- The Royal College of Speech and Language Therapists
- The Royal Pharmaceutical Society
- The Society of Chiropodists and Podiatrists.

Guidelines, clinical audit and care pathways are a useful means of getting the evidence into routine clinical practice. They are also helpful in managing and reducing the potential risks and in assessing feedback from complaints. These will be discussed in the next chapter.

References

1. Haynes B, Haines A 1998 Barriers and bridges to evidence based clinical practice. British Medical Journal 317: 273-276
2. Rosenberg W, Donald A 1995 Evidence based medicine: an approach to clinical problem solving. British Medical Journal 310(6987): 1122-1126
3. Sackett D L, Rosenberg W M C, Gray J A M et al 1996 Evidence based medicine: what it is and what it isn't. British Medical Journal 312: 71-72
4. Bero L A, Grilli R, Grimshaw J et al 1998 Closing the gap between research and practice: an overview of systematic reviews of interventions to promote the implementation of research findings British Medical Journal 317: 465-468
5. National Pathways Association 1998 Care pathways definition. NPA Newsletter, spring
6. Campbell H, Hotchkiss R, Bradshaw N et al 1998 Integrated care pathways. British Medical Journal 316: 133-137
7. Carins C, Shepherd G 1997 Pathways to the future for community diabetes care. In: Wilson J (ed) Integrated care management: the path to success? Butterworth-Heinemann, Oxford
8. Layton A, Moss F, Morgan G 1998 Mapping out the patient's journey: experiences of developing pathways of care. Quality in Healthcare 7 (suppl): S30-36
9. Department of Health 1989 Working for patients. HMSO, London
10. Department of Health 1994 Clinical audit in the nursing and therapy professions. HMSO, London
11. NHS Executive 1996 Promoting clinical effectiveness: a framework for action in and through the NHS. NHS Executive, London
12. Berkshire Medical Audit Advisory Group and Berkshire Health Authority 1998 County-wide interface stroke/TIA audit. Berkshire Medical Audit Advisory Group and Berkshire Health Authority, Reading
13. Cheater F M, Keane M 1998 Nurses' participation in audit: a regional study. Quality in Healthcare 7: 27-36
14. The National Centre for Clinical Audit 1997 Planning a clinical audit – a checklist for good practice. The National Centre for Clinical Audit, London
15. NHS Executive, London Region 1999 Clinical governance in London Region: draft template of clinical audit report for a Trust Board. http://www.doh.gov.uk/ntro/template.htm
16. NHS Executive 1997 Clinical effectiveness resource pack. HMSO, London

6

Complaints and risk management

Complaints

It is all too easy to perceive complaints by patients as negative and destructive feedback on the work of clinicians who, by and large, provide the best care they can. In such a large organisation as the NHS, which in reality is made up of smaller independent sub-units (PCTs, NHS trusts, independent contractors etc.), some systems and forms of health care delivery do fail, giving rise to dissatisfaction. Before 1996, the NHS complaints system itself exacerbated this discontent by being clumsy and lengthy, with the process having a strong association with disciplinary procedures. This situation was assessed by the review committee on NHS complaints procedures, chaired by Professor Alan Wilson, and a report, *Being Heard*, was published in 1994.[1] This was then developed by the Government into a revised policy on complaints, called *Acting on Complaints*,[2] which proposed the setting up of a new complaints procedure in 1996. The key objectives for the new procedure were to:[3]

- provide ease of access for patients and complainants
- provide a simplified procedure, with common features, for complaints about any of the services provided as part of the NHS
- separate complaints from disciplinary procedures
- make it easier to extract lessons on quality from complaints to improve services for patients
- be fair to staff and complainants alike
- provide a more rapid and open process
- provide an approach that is honest and thorough, with the main aim of resolving the problems and satisfying the concerns of the complainant.

Issues for consideration

- Some of the key objectives of the complaints procedure reflect some of the main objectives for clinical governance (e.g. learning lessons, improving the quality of care, and the process being open to scrutiny). What, in your organisation, have been some of the major lessons learnt from this process?
- If there has not been any feedback from this process in your organisation, why is this the case?

The complaints procedure is essentially split into two parts; local resolution and independent review.

Local resolution

The time scale allowed for receipt of the original complaint is 6 months from the event, or 6 months of becoming aware of the event, and no longer than 12 months. Complainants are defined as existing or former patients of the relevant trust, PCT or practice. Complaints can be made by those acting on behalf of the patient.

The emphasis is on resolving complaints as quickly as possible through an immediate local response. The time scales reflect this, with an acknowledgement required within 2 working days of receipt and full reply within 20 working days (10 days for practice-based complaints).

Front-line staff in any NHS organisation are at the initial receiving end of the complaint, and so should be appropriately trained to manage this type of situation and, where necessary, to recognise when to refer for a fuller investigation by or co-ordination through the complaints manager. Steps should also be taken by front-line staff to ensure that complainants are aware of the role of the Community Health Council and any other patients' advocates available to assist in pursuing complaints.

The NHS organisation must have a designated complaints manager who is readily accessible to the public and has an overall perspective of the complaints system. This person can be the Chief Executive, but is more usually a senior manager reporting directly to or with personal access to the Chief Executive in an NHS trust, PCT or, in general practice, a lead GP or practice manager. The complaints process also applies to the other independent contractor groups (i.e. dentists, high street pharmacists and optometrists).

In primary care, some situations may occur when a relationship has broken down between a patient and a GP to such an extent that there is a need for the intervention of conciliators. These are people appointed by or working for the PCT or the local representative committees (i.e. local

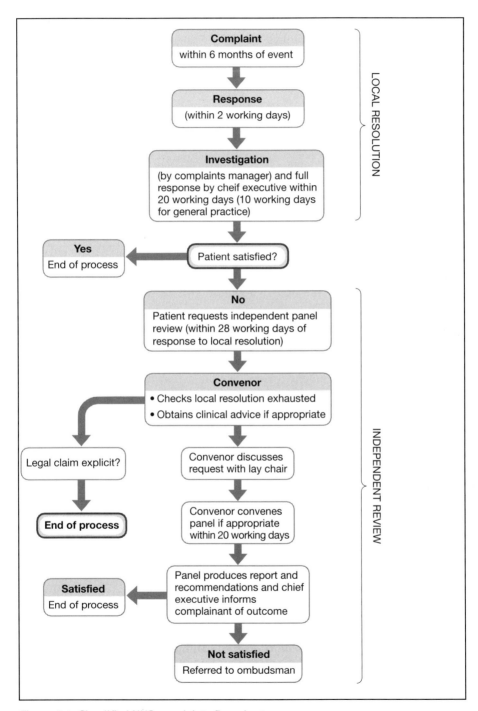

Figure 6.1 Simplified NHS complaints flow chart

medical committee, local dental committee, local pharmaceutical committee or local optical committee), whose task is to bring together the two parties to discuss and resolve the complaint. This process can be used as an intermediate step to settle the complaint without recourse to an independent review.

It is important to make a note of the circumstances of the complaint as close to the event as possible, while the memories are still fresh. All responses to written complaints should also be in writing by the Chief Executive or lead GP.

Above all, it is important that the patient who requires health care continues to receives this.

Independent review

If a complainant feels that the matter has not been resolved satisfactorily using local resolution, they do have a right to request an independent review from the trust or the PCT's convenor. This request must be made within 28 calendar days from the completion of the local resolution process, and the information supporting this must be obtained in a statement signed by the complainant.

The role of convenor of a PCT or NHS trust is to consider the requests by complainants for independent review. The main task is to ensure that the local resolution process has been adequately followed before the need to set up a review panel is considered. The convenor should not have had any previous involvement in the complaint at the local resolution stage, as this could possibly affect their judgement.

The convenor discusses the request with an independent lay panel chair, who is nominated by the Secretary of State for Health. The purpose of this is to provide an external independent view and to aid in the assessment of the complaint. Where the complaint involves clinical judgement, the convenor needs to take appropriate clinical advice. However, it is the convenor who decides whether or not to set up an independent panel and explains the decision. The response to the request for the independent review should be made within 20 working days.

The following criteria should be exhausted before an independent review panel is established:

- Whether any other action, short of establishing a panel should be taken
- If all practical action has been taken, in which case establishing a panel will not add any further value.

The independent review panel consists of three members; a lay chair, the convenor of the relevant PCT or NHS trust, and a representative of the purchaser (for NHS trusts) or another independent person (for a PCT). If the complaint is a clinical complaint, the panel is advised by at least two independent clinical assessors, nominated by the strategic health authority, following advice from the relevant professional bodies.

The function of the panel is to investigate the aspects of the complaint stated in the terms of reference set out by the convenor, and to make a report with conclusions and, if appropriate, recommendations. The report is sent to the following:[3]

- the complainant
- the patient, if a different person from the complainant and competent to receive the report
- any person named in the complaint
- any person interviewed by the panel
- the clinical assessors
- the NHS trust/PCT authority chair and Chief Executive
- the GP/dentist/pharmacist/optometrist concerned, if it is this type of complaint
- the strategic health authority
- the PCT chair and Chief Executive who purchased the service concerned.

The report should be presented to the board of the PCT or NHS trust concerned for discussion and for action to be taken as a result of the complaint. The complainant should be informed of the outcome of this process by the Chief Executive, and also of the right to take their grievance to the ombudsman (Health Service Commissioner).

Referral to the ombudsman is a last resort, and investigation will only occur if:

- the complaint is not investigated by the relevant NHS organisation because it fell outside the NHS time limits
- the complainant is dissatisfied following local resolution and the convenor has refused a request for an independent review
- the complainant is dissatisfied with the process or the outcome of the independent review.

If a complaint reveals a case of negligence, or if it is thought that there is a likelihood of legal action, then this becomes a risk management matter and should be referred to the person responsible for dealing with this area within the NHS trust or PCT.

At the time of writing the complaints procedure is under review and the bodies dealing with the local resolution and independent review may change.

Some examples of complaints

A 68-year-old man with a long history of stomach ulcers presented to A&E with abdominal pain, and treatment for a perforated ulcer was given. Three months later the man complained of severe abdominal pain, and was booked in for an urgent gastroscopy and ultrasound examination. Before the appointment was due the man presented to A&E again with abdominal pain, and some non-absorbable suture material was found from the previous surgery. Following treatment, the man was discharged but no outpatient appointment was given. The man's condition deteriorated again; he was admitted as an emergency and investigation revealed that he had a deep abscess. He was booked for surgery. This was delayed, however, due to a full operating list. Following the operation the man was discharged on a Friday evening and told to go to his GP for further medication on the Monday. The man died three months later. The man's wife complained that there was insufficient communication by the hospital staff about his condition, and there was poor follow-up after discharge. The hospital found that the hospital notes were patchy and it was difficult to obtain the full picture from them.

An 84-year-old woman with a history of chronic asthma was admitted to hospital with severe breathlessness. This was treated, as was another chest infection, which extended her stay. Two days after discharge, the woman's condition deteriorated suddenly and she died on her way to hospital. The GP put on the death certificate that the cause was bronchopneumonia. Her daughter complained that her mother's condition was insufficiently treated and that she was discharged too early. The hospital records, however, indicated that the infection was treated appropriately. The independent panel could not uphold the complaint, saying that the clinical assessors suggested that she could have died of a heart attack.

A 34-year-old woman with a long history of irritable bowel syndrome presented to her GP with abdominal pain. The GP gave her the usual treatment for this condition. The woman phoned the GP 3 hours later, saying that the pain had worsened, and requested a visit. The GP did not visit, and the woman eventually went to A&E as her pain had worsened. She was found to have an ectopic pregnancy, which was treated. The woman's husband complained that the GP had failed to visit his wife. The GP said that the woman was a difficult patient and he had often been called out to visit her for her irritable bowel syndrome.

The survey carried out by the Medical Defence Union in the first year of the complaints procedure in 1996/97[4] revealed the following causes of the complaints to GPs and highlighted the importance of local resolution in the process (see Table 6.1).

Table 6.1 Survey carried out by Medical Defence Union[4]

Cause for complaint	Percentage
Failure/delay in diagnosis	32
Inadequate treatment/management	22
Attitude or rudeness of doctor	11
Failure/delay to visit	8
Failure/delay to refer	5
Prescription error	4
Breach of confidentiality	4
Administration	2
Communication	2
Other	10

An analysis of the GP complaints procedure in its first year (1996/97) by the Medical Defence Union[4]

- Of the 558 GP complaints notified to the MDU in the first 9 months of the new procedure, 81% were resolved at local resolution
- 3.5% of complainants indicated that they were proceeding to a claim of alleged negligence *
- 0.5% of complaints resulted in a referral to the GMC *
- 13% of complaints had proceeded (or may proceed) to independent review
- 2% of the total requested independent review and were declined and referred back for local resolution
- No complaints were referred to the ombudsman
- 23% of complaints were made following a bereavement
- GP co-operatives have an increased chance for failure/delay to visit, but these had been resolved locally.

* = equivalent to a similar study carried out by the MDU on complaints in 1995.

Apart from the specific causes for complaining as highlighted in the MDU study, people complain for other reasons. Bark and colleagues[5] found, in their study of complainants, the following reasons for complaining about health services:

- so that this type of incident will not happen again
- to raise the awareness of staff concerning the problems
- to get an explanation of what went wrong
- to receive an apology for the incident
- to discipline the relevant staff responsible for the care

- to obtain further clinical treatment
- to get compensation.

There was, in the study, a tenfold difference in ranking between the first and last reason given for complaints, highlighting the fact that monetary gain is not a major factor in people making complaints. However, complaints are on the same continuum as clinical risk, near misses and adverse incidents, and they should not be seen as minor events compared to negligence. An unsatisfactory answer to a complaint at whatever level can easily become a claim for compensation for the wrong reasons.

The motivation for coming clean about clinical incidents is even harder for staff, especially if patients have adverse experiences as a result of treatment. For example, in the same study, the researchers found that half of the complainants required further treatment; the patient's condition had deteriorated as a result of treatment in 40% of cases, and a third experienced side effects. In addition 5% of complaints were made by bereaved relatives.

Issues for consideration

- Has the complaints department produced a summary of complaints dealt with by your organisation?
- If so, has there been any note of the recommendations made or other action required?
- What specific improvements in services have you personally been involved in following issues raised by the complaints procedure?

An important feature in the management of complaints is to recognise the effect a complaint has on those who are on the receiving end of it. A response to a complaint must also deal with the individual member of staff's reaction. If this not managed well, there is a danger of fuelling the dissatisfaction. Common (and not unexpected) reactions to complaints include:[6]

- anger
- defensiveness
- confusion
- distress
- resentment
- guilt
- concern for the patient if harm has been done
- a feeling of personal failure
- great stress

- loss of confidence
- shame.

The reactions need an opportunity for airing before any meeting with the complainant occurs in order to avoid a confrontational outcome. Other support to staff faced with this situation can include:[6]

- counselling
- support from management
- support from colleagues
- support groups for this purpose
- a help line
- regular feedback on the progress of a case
- quality legal advice where necessary
- identification of the contributing events that led to the complaint
- training in effective handling of complaints
- training in communication and interpersonal skills.

These reactions, as well as understanding the agenda (i.e. why the patient has complained), are vital to the process of learning from the complaint in order to act appropriately.

The tackling of complaints close to the point and time of the incident occurring provides an opportunity to 'nip things in the bud' and to resolve the situation satisfactorily. The challenge, now, is for clinical governance to pick out the salient features of the lessons learnt from the process as highlighted by Bark's study, in addition to the individual cases occurring at NHS organisation level, and to channel this into improvements in service delivery and clinical care.

Risk management

Consider the following situations:

1. Over the course of 2 months in 1991, a number of children in a paediatric ward collapsed unexpectedly and died after seeming to be on a course of recovery from their illnesses. These events were noticed by the hospital staff, but no action was taken initially. It was only when a grossly abnormal insulin level was detected in one child that criminal behaviour was considered. Subsequently, in a review of the X-rays of two of the children who survived, one had evidence of rib fractures which appeared to be the result of violence and the other had evidence of air having been deliberately injected into the arm and axilla. Eventually, a young and inexperienced nurse called Beverly Allitt was

found to be the cause of the unexplained deaths. A report into the events concluded that no single individual could be held responsible for what had happened, but if there had been a system to detect such activity and there had been a discussion amongst the various health professionals involved, the number of deaths could have been reduced or even prevented.[7]

2. In a tertiary centre in Bristol, in the 1980s and early 1990s, the mortality rates for babies undergoing complex cardiac operations were noted to be high. Nothing was done to investigate this, and the surgeons in the unit continued to operate. Events came to a head when, in 1995, an 18-month-old boy died on the operating table. In 1998 the General Medical Council struck off one of the cardiac surgeons responsible and the Chief Executive, who was also a doctor, and disciplined the second cardiac surgeon.

In both examples, the two root causes were:

- a failure in the systems within the organisations and related agencies to alert the authorities to the adverse incidents occurring
- a failure to respond quickly when the trends were noticed.

In any situation in life there is risk, and health care is no exception. However, steps can be taken to minimise risk by putting systems in place to document and monitor clinical care.

Definition of risk

the possibility of incurring misfortune or loss (Collins Dictionary)
the potential for unwanted outcome (Wilson,1994[8])
This misfortune results in:

- harm to patients
- resources being diverted to provide extra treatment to correct the initial injury
- resources diverted to the investigation of complaints, adverse incidents and medical negligence
- harm to the reputation of the provider because of poor performance
- a reduction of public confidence in the provider concerned.

Risk is a part of everyday life and so the aim is to minimise its effect through appropriate risk management. Risk management, and in particular clinical risk management, is an area which has been reasonably well developed within the health service in specific sectors and specialties. The driving force has been the escalating claims for medical negligence, which rise rapidly year on year, and is a reflection of the increased volume of NHS activity, a growing trend for patients to seek redress when incidents occur, and upward pressures on the size of negligence awards greatly exceeding the general level of litigation.[9] The main effect of rising litigation is that increasing resources are being diverted to settle clinical negligence claims, and these could otherwise have been used for patient care.

Cost of litigation[9]	
1990/91	£53m
1993/94	£125m
1994/95	£150m
1995/96	£200m
1996/97	£300m[10]
1999/2000	£386m[11]

At the time of writing the total liability (i.e. the cumulative cost of litigation to the NHS) is estimated to be £4.4bn.[12]

Risk management systems incorporate a number of related processes, which include complaints and medical negligence, as shown below:

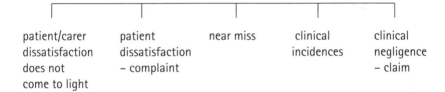

| patient/carer dissatisfaction does not come to light | patient dissatisfaction – complaint | near miss | clinical incidences | clinical negligence – claim |

A definition of risk management[13]
A means of reducing the risks of adverse events occurring in organisations by systematically assessing, reviewing and then seeking ways to prevent their occurrence. Clinical risk management takes place in a clinical setting.

A simple way of looking at risk management is to get things right the first time – in other words, to change the environment whereby the systems and behaviours can be modified to reduce the potential for health care risk. Although there are some specialties that have a greater risk than others, there are generic causes of risk that can be applied to any health care setting.

Specialties with a high risk[14]

- Accident and emergency *
- Anaesthetics *
- General surgery *
- Gynaecology *
- General medicine
- Paediatrics
- Obstetrics *
- Cardiac surgery
- Orthopaedics *

* specialties at greatest risk

Reasons why unnecessary risks occur[14]

- System failures (e.g. ill-defined, or the lack of appropriate, processes, policies, procedures and clinical guidelines)
- Staff taking short cuts due to heavy workload, pressures of work and lack of support
- Breakdown of communication between a number of parties (e.g. health care professionals, patients, carers) and different agencies
- Ill-defined responsibilities (e.g. roles are unclear or exceeding the scope of individual staff skills and competencies)
- Inadequately trained staff
- Poor co-ordination of care in teams or between agencies
- Deliberate damage to patients by staff.

Example

An 83-year-old woman was admitted to hospital in a confused state. On the day after her admission, nurses found her bed empty. She was eventually found in the linen cupboard standing on top of a mattress, trying to get to the window. After this, the nurses requested a window restraint for the ward, which had none at the time. When the carpenter came to assess the windows, it became clear that all of the windows needed restraints and he had to go away and make them. At noon the same day, a nurse waiting in the grounds for a bus looked up and saw the patient falling out of a window. Ten years prior to the incident in 1989, guidelines had been issued to all trusts recommending that all window restraints and electric doors be fitted for all wards housing vulnerable or confused patients. The hospital had no risk assessment system in place, and was fined nearly £16,500 for breaching the Health and Safety at Work Act.

Definition of a clinical incident[15]

An unexpected event occurring during treatment, or unexpected result of treatment, which may, or does, cause harm to the patient.

Definition of a near miss[14]

An occurrence which, but for luck or skilful management, would in all probability have become an incident.

The reporting of these events requires the nurturing of an open, honest and blame-free culture within an organisation.

Risk management strategy

The approach to managing risk is to develop a strategy following four key steps.[14] This must also be in the context of the overall clinical governance strategy.

Table 6.2 Risk management strategy[14]

1. Risk identification

This is the awareness of risk by the organisation. Many sources can be used to identify potential risk, including incident reporting, which is an important feature in this process. Early identification of near misses, incidents and other mistakes will lead to effective risk management.

2. Risk analysis

This is an assessment of the potential severity of the loss associated with an identified risk and the probability that such a loss will occur. An effective complaints and claims management system is an important component of such an analysis.

3. Risk treatment

This refers to the range of choices available in handling a given risk. It includes:
● risk control – control measures to contain risks, reducing the likelihood of an adverse occurrence or outcome (e.g. guidelines, education and training, contingency or disaster planning etc.)
● risk acceptance – this involves managing a risk that cannot be otherwise reduced, transferred or avoided; here, an assumption is made of the potential losses associated with a given risk, making plans to cover any financial consequences of such a loss (e.g. the demand for a new expensive treatment or intervention that is clinically effective)
● risk avoidance – this is the use of alternative ways of providing care, which reduces the greater risk posed by the original method

- risk reduction or minimisation – this is at the heart of most health care organisation risk management programmes, and includes activities such as staff education and training, policy and procedure revision etc.
- risk transfer – this involves shifting the risk of loss to other entities (e.g. by a pooling arrangement with other organisations such as the Central Negligence Scheme for Trusts or the Welsh Risk Pool)

4. Evaluation of risk treatment strategies

This is the multidisciplinary approach to reviewing and evaluating the effectiveness of the risk management programme.

One tool that can be used in the identification and management of risk is the care pathway (see Chapter 5).

Issues for consideration

Consider a risk in your workplace or in the clinical care of patients.

- What action was taken to tackle the risk?
- What lessons were learnt from that process?

The Central Negligence Scheme For Trusts was set up in 1995, with the aim of facilitating the planning for very large claims (or a run of high claims or serial claims) through the provision of financial assistance. Trusts contribute to a pool from which the claims can be paid, and in turn receive financial support according to the level of standards they achieve in managing risk within their organisations.

Ten standards have now been developed[16] with a separate set of standards for maternity services.[17]

1. Learning from experience
2. Response to major clinical incidents
3. Advice and consent
4. Health records
5. Induction, training and competence
6. Implementation of clinical risk management
7. Clinical care
8. The management of care in trusts providing mental health services
9. Ambulance service
10. Maternity care.[17]

Trusts are assessed, at least once every two years, against the first 7 'core' standards, with additional standards for the trusts providing mental health care, ambulance services and maternity care. Each of the standards have a number of criteria against which trusts can be assessed in order to define a level of compliance, at level 1, 2 or full compliance, 3. The higher the level, the greater the discount trusts can receive on their contribution to the scheme.

Similar schemes are available from the Welsh Risk Pool in Wales and the Clinical Negligence and Other Risks Indemnity Scheme in Scotland.

An additional risk for NHS organisations is the effect of the changes imposed by the report *Access to Justice* (the Woolf report),[18] in which civil action cases are dealt with in short specified time scales to speed up the claims process. If the time scales are not met, trusts are subject to severe penalties. Early identification of potential claims and accurate reporting from everyone involved in an incident at the time are essential risk strategies to meet these obligations.

Examples of changes in clinical practice arising from clinical risk management[19]

- Use of bed rails and other measures to prevent falls
- Equipment and arrangements for manual handling improved
- Introduction of pre-operative clinics
- Consent practice changed
- Guidance issues on managing/using syringe drivers
- New prescription sheets introduced
- Management of suspected aortic aneurysms in A&E changed
- Reduction in the use of mercury thermometers
- Specimen labelling and transport tightened up
- Swab counting procedure in theatre improved
- Policy on use of heparin introduced
- Procedure used for female sterilisation changed
- Syringes labelled when drugs drawn up but not used immediately
- Cardiopulmonary resuscitation trolleys audited regularly
- Development of patient information leaflets that cite risks as well as benefits
- Theatre booking changed – more evenly spaced, enabling better use
- Development of new policy for managing serious untoward events.

Risk management strategy for child protection (South Warwickshire Combined Care NHS Trust)

1. Child protection information
A clear system for identifying the numbers of children on the child protection register
A clear system to identify the children about whom there are concerns by health professionals

2. Child protection supervision
One-to-one child protection supervision for health visitors
Ad hoc supervision as the need arises, accessible to all health professionals

3. Policies/guidelines
Warwickshire-wide policies are in use within the trust

4. Documentation
A letter format for confirmation of verbal child protection referral is in use
Report forms for child protection case conferences/reviews are in use
Report forms for supervision meeting with clinical leaders are in use

5. Training
Approved child area protection committee level 1 child protection training is provided for all staff who may have contact with children during the course of their work
Update training is available on an annual basis, plus training to specific professional groups as requested
There is a 10 minute child protection slot in the trust induction course to inform new staff of the child protection procedures.

In a survey of their trusts and general practices in 1998, the North Thames Region found that clinical risk management was at an embryonic stage of development.[20]

Table 6.3 Survey of Trusts and General Practices 1998[20]

Trusts

The survey found that:
A risk management system was in place in 90% of trusts, but was only introduced on average over the last 22 months
48% of trusts are using software to analyse trends
80% of trusts are linking risk management to their complaints procedure
Only 56% of trusts had arranged specific training for their staff
Only 25% of trusts had provided a report for their board

General practices

The survey found that:
51% of practices are using some form of risk management
54% of practices do some trend analysis of complaints
49% of practices have set up a critical incident reporting system
62% of practices undertake random prescribing checks
35% of practices have a health and safety manual, and those that do not would like one

From the findings of the survey, the London Regional Office of the NHS Executive developed a template of audit of risk management for use by trust boards to monitor the progress of the process.[13] Four main components of a risk management approach are highlighted (the full template is in the toolkit at the end of the book):

- The risk management system with the right culture
- Current use of the system
- Impact on patient care
- Value for money.

Using the audit template, a suggested report for submission to the trust board was proposed:[13]

1. Introduction
2. Structures
   - staff support
   - risk management committee
   - clinical claims review group
   - local risk management groups
   - *ad hoc* investigation panels
3. Education and training for staff
   - risk management
   - complaints
   - complaints reporting
4. Adverse incident reporting
   - process and database
   - feedback of incident data
   - overview of data held on database
   - data quality
   - in-depth reviews; rolling programme
5. Links with clinical governance
   - risk management involvement in other corporate groups
6. Claims
   - expert advice and support
   - clinical claims review group
   - claims profile
   - CNST standards (see toolkit)
7. Improvements, new policies and actions
   - risk management
   - complaints
8. Costs
   - staffing

- claims/legal/CNST costs
9. Action plan summary for the year
  - current position
  - future development of risk management.

The national patient safety agency

In 1999 a report called *An Organisation with a Memory* was produced by an expert committee chaired by the Chief Medical Officer, Professor Liam Donaldson.[21] It examined the size, nature and causes of the problem of avoidable failures in service in the NHS, assessed the experience, research and good practice from other areas outside of health on operational failures, proposed the best methods of identifying problems (including the collection and analysis of data) and made some recommendations as to the best approach for making improvements.

The report identified a number of areas where the NHS has paid a high price for failure:[21]

- 400 people died or were seriously injured in adverse events involving medical devices as reported to the Medical Devices Agency in 1999
- Nearly 10,000 people were reported to have experienced serious adverse reactions to drugs
- Around 1,150 people who had been in recent contact with mental health services committed suicide
- Nearly 28,000 written complaints about aspects of clinical treatment in hospitals, and over 38,000 complaints about family health services, were made in 1998/99
- The NHS paid out around £400 million as settlement for clinical negligence claims in 1998/99, and had a potential liability of around £2.4 billion for existing and expected claims. When the claims were analysed, many of the cases had potentially avoidable causes
- Hospital acquired infections, around 15% of which may be regarded as preventable, were estimated to cost the NHS nearly £1 billion a year.

The report made ten recommendations:

An organisation with a memory – recommendations[21]

1. Introduce a mandatory reporting scheme for adverse health care events and specified near misses
2. Introduce a scheme for confidential reporting by staff of adverse events and near misses

3. Encourage a reporting and questioning culture in the NHS
4. Introduce a single overall system for analysing and disseminating lessons from adverse health care events and near misses
5. Make better use of existing sources of information on adverse events
6. Improve the quality and relevance of NHS adverse event investigations and inquiries
7. Undertake a programme of basic research into adverse health care events in the NHS
8. Make full use of new NHS information systems to help staff access learning from adverse health care events and near misses
9. Act to ensure that important lessons are implemented quickly and consistently
10. Identify and address specific categories of serious recurring adverse health care event.

Building a safer NHS for patients

The Government's response to *An Organisation with a Memory* was the implementation document, *Building a Safer NHS for Patients*[22] in which a number of recommended actions were identified for the NHS in England.

Recommendations of *Building a Safer NHS for Patients*[22]

- The establishment of a mandatory, national reporting scheme for adverse health care events
- The setting up of a new National Patient Safety Agency
- The setting up of a new system for handling investigations and inquiries across the NHS
- The following four specific areas of risk were to be targeted for action:
  - to reduce to zero the number of patients killed or paralysed by maladministered spinal injections by December 2001
  - to reduce by 25% the number of instances of harm in obstetrics and gynaecology which lead to litigation by the end of 2005
  - to reduce by 40% the number of serious errors in the use of prescribed drugs by the end of 2005
  - to reduce to zero the number of suicides by mental health patients as a consequence of hanging from non-collapsible bed or shower curtain rails on wards by March 2002
- The development of a strategy for patient safety research to improve understanding of the underlying causes of why things go wrong.

The cornerstone of *Building a Safer NHS for Patients* was the establishment of the National Patient Safety Agency, which started its work in July 2001.

Its role is to implement the recommendations which have been identified in the paper; in particular, the development of a national reporting system for the recording of adverse health care events.

The agency's role is:[23]

- to set and maintain standards for reporting for the NHS
- to collect, collate, categorise and code adverse event information from the NHS
- to gather other safety-related information from other sources
- to analyse information and maintain records which will be available to the public
- to provide feedback on the main issues identified and key lessons learned from the reporting system to organisations and individuals
- to produce solutions to reduce risk and prevent harm for future patients
- to set national goals and targets on reducing risk and harm prevention
- to promote research on patient safety
- to promote a reporting culture within the NHS which is supportive and constructive
- to collaborate with other bodies.

The reporting system has the following key principles:

- it is mandatory for both individuals and NHS organisations
- it is confidential, but open and accessible
- it is generally free of blame and independent
- it should be simple to use, but must be comprehensive in coverage and in the type of data collected
- it will encourage and develop systems for learning and change at both local and national levels.

The type of information that needs to be recorded for adverse events and near misses is defined as follows:[23]

- What happened?
- Where did it happen?
- When did it happen?
- How did it happen?
- Why did it happen?
- What action was taken or proposed?
- What impact did the event have?
- What factors did, or could have, minimised the impact of the event?

Record keeping

The effective management of complaints and clinical risk, and indeed good clinical care, is very much dependent on accurate and legible record keeping. Poorly written records make it very difficult to defend medical negligence cases if they are unclear or not easy to understand. The Audit Commission[24] reported some serious shortcomings in medical record keeping in hospitals. They noted the following problems:

- 30% of history sheets were inadequate – illegible, not dated, timed or signed
- 40% of handwritten discharge medication sheets were illegible
- 80% of medical records did not have a patient identified on every piece of paper relating to that patient
- 40% of records were badly kept or not updated
- 50% of records had no index of their contents on the front
- 90% of discharge summaries had no reference to any information given to patient or to their relatives.

Example

A diabetic man underwent an operation for vascular surgery, which was successful. A care plan was devised for his time spent in the recovery room, covering regular 15-minute observations on temperature, pulse and blood pressure and leg sensation. At one point the records cease and do not begin again until 2^{1}/2 hours later, when there was a difficulty in obtaining a reading for blood pressure. However, 10 minutes later the reading was recorded as 120/80. Despite this, 5 minutes later the man had a cardiac arrest; he was returned to theatre and died an hour later.

The messages gleaned from complaints and risk management need to be identified and fed back to staff. The audit process and the use of care pathways as described in Chapter 5 are two methods of feedback. Another process is through the education and training route, which addresses the requirement for the professional development of clinicians. The various approaches to education, training and professional development will be described in Chapter 7.

References
1. Department of Health 1994 'Being heard': report of the review committee on NHS complaints procedures, chaired by Professor Alan Wilson. HMSO, London

2. Department of Health 1995 Acting on complaints: the Government's proposals. HMSO, London

3. NHS Executive 1996 Complaints: listening... acting... improving. Guidance on implementation of the NHS complaints procedure. NHS Executive, London

4. Green S, Price J 1997 New complaints procedure: exclusive MDU report of first year. Pulse 5th April: 56-65

5. Bark P, Vincent C, Jones A et al 1994 Clinical complaints: a means of improving quality of care. Quality in Healthcare 3: 123-132

6. Bark P 1999 Complaints: the carer's perspective. In: Wilson J, Tingle J (eds) Clinical risk modification, a route to clinical governance? Butterworth-Heinemann, Oxford

7. Report of the independent inquiry relating to deaths and injuries on the children's ward at Grantham and Kesteven General Hospital during the period February to April 1991, chaired by Sir Cecil Clothier. HMSO, London

8. Wilson J H 1994 Quality in clinical care, healthcare risk modification. Health Business Summary, April

9. Department of Health 1996 Clinical negligence costs. FDL 96: 39

10. Hansard 1998 House of Commons debate for 24 March, column 165. The Stationery Office, London

11. Key facts. http://www.nhsla.com

12. National Audit Office 2002 NHS summarised accounts 2000-01. http://www.nao.gov.uk

13. NHS Executive, London Region 1999 Clinical governance in London Region: draft template of audit risk management report for a Trust Board. http://www.doh.gov.uk/ntro/risktemp.htm

14. Wilson J H 1999 Risk reviews and using a risk management strategy. In: Wilson J, Tingle J (eds) Clinical risk modification, a route to clinical governance? Butterworth Heinemann, Oxford

15. Pincombe C 1995 The clinical negligence scheme for trusts. Risk management – a new approach (2). Clinical Risk 1(3): 132-134

16. NHS Litigation Authority 2002 Clinical risk management standards. NHS Litigaition Authority, London

17. Clinical Negligence Scheme for Trusts 2002 Clinical risk management standards for maternity services, draft 4. NHS Litigation Authority and Clinical Negligence Scheme for Trusts, London

18. Lord Woolf 1996 Access to justice: final report. HMSO, London

19. Walshe K, Dineen M 1998 Risky business. Health Management October: 14-15

20. NHS Executive, North Thames Region 1998 Clinical governance in North Thames: a paper for discussion and consultation. NHS Executive North Thames Region, London

21. Expert Group on Learning from Adverse Events in the NHS 2000 An organisation with a memory. The Stationery Office, London http://www.doh.gov.uk/orgmemreport/index.htm

22. Department of Health 2001 Building a safer NHS for patients. The Stationery Office, London http://www.doh.gov.uk/buildsafnhs

23. Department of Health 2000 Building a safer NHS for patients: briefing. NHS Confederation Publications, London
24. The Audit Commission 1995 Setting the records straight: a study of hospital medical records. HMSO, London

7

Support for clinical governance

The support for clinical governance involves two main areas; the training and development of clinical and non-clinical staff to ensure the delivery of health care, and timely and accurate information on which to base clinical decisions and monitor performance and outcomes. This chapter provides an overall perspective on how these two fit in with the duty of clinical governance. For more extensive discussions of these areas, the reader is referred to detailed, expert texts in the relevant subjects.

Continuous professional development

The White Paper *A First Class Service*,[1] envisages lifelong learning and continuous professional development (CPD) as an essential component in the development of clinical governance. In order for health professionals to provide effective care, they need to make sure that their own skills, knowledge and expertise are up-to-date. Although there had been a fair amount of CPD activity in a number of professions prior to the establishment of clinical governance, few links were made between this and clinical effectiveness and research and development. The aim of CPD is to match the legitimate aspirations of individual health professionals and to respond to service development and patient expectations. The essential process is that this should be developed on a local level within every health organisation. The importance of CPD has been highlighted by the fact that it was one of the first targets in the establishment of clinical governance in the NHS.

What is lifelong learning?

Lifelong learning:[2]
Aims to ensure that all health care staff have the up-to-date skills and knowledge required to deliver high quality care. Effective lifelong learning depends on every health organisation developing its learning environment. As part of this, every health organisation needs to have a locally managed system of continuing professional development with the emphasis on learning in teams and more work-based learning. Investment in CPD programmes needs to match local health care objectives and should link with other developments in the NHS, providing a more effective and integrated approach to lifelong learning.

What is continuous professional development?

Continuous professional development is:[3]
An individual taking responsibility for the development of his/her own career by systematically analysing development needs, identifying and using appropriate methods to meet these needs and regularly reviewing achievement compared against personal and career objectives.

Continuous professional development programmes are best managed locally, and follow a circular pathway.[1]

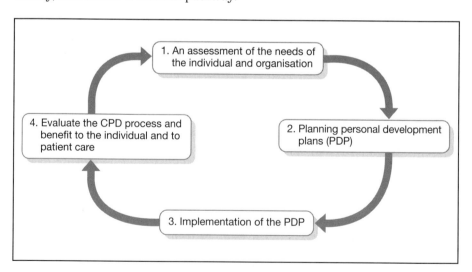

Figure 7.1 Continuous professional development programme following a circular pathway. From *A First Class Service: Quality in the New NHS*[1]

For CPD to be successful for an individual, there needs to be a clear understanding of the way in which that individual learns and develops most effectively. There are several well-documented learning theories. The two theories most widely referred to are the analyses of Kolb's four learning styles, and Honey and Mumford's four learning types, which followed some 12 years later.[4] Both these analyses have an accompanying questionnaire that will give individuals some insight into their preferred learning style and some ideas on how they can experiment with an alternative approach.

Identifying learning needs

An educational researcher, Knowles,[5] developed the following structure for the identification of the learning needs of an individual and how the learning objectives could be evaluated once specified and implemented:

1. Diagnose the learning needs
   - Assess the gap between where the individual is now and where he/she wants to be.
   - Specify the areas requiring most attention, concentrating on what is liked and disliked.

2. Specify learning objectives
   - How will the learning needs be met?
   - The objectives should state the level of competency that is desired, and should be achievable in realistic time scales.
   - The objectives can either relate to the individual's internal development or to some change in behaviour. Examples include:
     - clinical knowledge and skills
     - medico-political and legal knowledge
     - quality assessment and audit
     - management and administration
     - information, management and technology
     - interpersonal skills/dealing with people.

3. Specify the learning resources and strategies
   - Consider the information requirements needed (sources of information are discussed in Chapter 4).

4. Specify evidence of accomplishment
   - The indicators could range from:
     - greater knowledge (e.g. on a specific subject)
     - better understanding

- acquisition of skills (e.g. critical appraisal skills – see Chapter 4)
- a change in attitude (e.g. a different approach to dealing with patients or carers)
- elucidation or acknowledgement of values

5. Specify how the evidence will be validated, i.e. how the learning objectives have been achieved – this can be demonstrated through a number of ways.

Validating the evidence

CPD can constitute a large list of activities, including:
- assessment/review of goals, objectives and tasks with a manager in a formal annual individual performance appraisal
- drawing up a personal development plan for the coming year
- peer review, formally or informally (e.g. GP appraisal)
- attending courses, conferences, study days, events, programmes
- formal qualifications, higher degrees
- secondment
- research/project work
- visits to other organisations
- a learning diary, to include, for example, significant event analysis
- being a member of a learning set
- having a mentor
- attending an assessment centre
- shadowing other people
- joining organisations (professional, managerial etc.) and attending events
- reading – books, journals etc.
- library club
- management or journal club
- networking
- career advice, help lines
- preparing for teaching and teaching itself
- writing for publication.

One of the main methods of formalising learning objectives and monitoring learning needs is to draw up a personal development plan (PDP).

Issues for consideration

- What is the approach of your organisation to CPD?
- Is it supportive or not?

- What are the opportunities available and the barriers to your carrying out CPD?

Table 7.1 Example of standards relating to CPD[6]

AUDIT FRAMEWORK

Target:	100%	
Exception:	2.	Not a mentoring system in place.
	4.	Lack of resources for agreed training needs.
Monitoring Method:	1. & 2.	Evidence of self evaluation and reflection of practice eg portfolio, professional development plan in place.
	3.	Review of documented evidence of outcome criteria.
	4.	Documented audit and research reports/results.
	5.	Named mentor available; mentoring system in place.
	6.	Dietitians training needs are documented and reported.
	7.	Audit in practice.
		Monitoring Examples 2a and 2b
References:	⇒	The British Dietetic Association *Towards the 21st Century Education & Training Strategy*, 1992
	⇒	The British Dietetic Association *Professional Portfolio*, 1994
	⇒	The British Dietetic Association *Advanced Diploma in Dietetic Practice*, 1995
	⇒	The British Dietetic Association *Mentoring in the Profession* (under development)
	⇒	Truelove S, *Handbook of Training and Development* (1992) Blackwell
	⇒	Institute of Personal Management, *Statement on Continuous Development – People and Work* (1987) EL 96/3
		Bound D, Cohen R & Walker D, (Eds), (1993), *Using Experience for Learning*, Buckingham, The Society for Research into Higher Education and Open University Press.
	⇒	Critten P, (1995), *Developing Your Portfolio*, London, Churchill Livingstone
	⇒	Down S, (1995), *Learning at Work: Making Things Happen*, London, Kogan Page.
	⇒	Schon D, (1983), *The Reflective Practitioner. How Professionals Think in Action*, New York Basic Books.
Implementation Date:		
Review Date:		

CONTINUING COMPETENCE TO PRACTICE

RATIONALE

Good professional practice requires up-to-date practitioners. Dietitians should be accountable for their own self-development and be responsible for identifying their ongoing continuous professional development (CPD) requirements. They must continue to improve their knowledge and develop their skills, through a process of self-evaluation and reflection on practice, in order to stay fit to practise in their specific areas. This includes attending courses, undertaking literature reviews, attending local meetings, learning from other colleagues. They need to recognise their own personal limitations. A framework is needed that links the Dietitian's personal and professional development with the objectives of the organisation in which they work. This must also address means of appraisal and how the agreed training needs are to be met.

STANDARD STATEMENT

Dietitians engage in self development to improve knowledge and skills in order to remain competent to practise within a framework which will include a suitable learning environment and appraisal system.

PROCESS CRITERIA	OUTCOME CRITERIA
1. The Dietitian will improve their knowledge and develop skills through a process of self-evaluation and reflection on practice.	1. There is written evidence which demonstrates that an assessment of the learning acquired has taken place.
2. The Dietitian will identify and record engagement in CPD activity.	2. There is written evidence of personal development plans: • professional portfolios • individual performance review.
3. The Dietitian will select CPD activities which enhance professional competence.	3. There is evidence that the Dietitian engages in informal learning through: • membership of BDA • membership of a BDA Special Interest Group • membership of other appropriate groups • reflection on day to day practice • reading journals and research papers • in-service training programmes • attending journal clubs • work shadowing • self directed learning • the supervision of student Dietitians.

cont/ . . .

3. The Dietitian will select CPD activities which enhance professional competence.	3. There is evidence that the Dietitian engages in formal learning through: • courses leading to degree or higher degree • post-registration qualifications eg BDA validated courses • participation in the Diploma in Advanced Dietetic Practice • undertaking research and presentation of work • attendance at conferences and seminars.
4. The Dietitian will be involved in agreed research and audit projects as appropriate to their post.	4. There is evidence: • of published audit and research • that current information and research is incorporated into dietetic practice at a local level.
5. The Dietitian will be involved in and understands the mentoring process.	5. There is evidence that the Dietitian has access to a mentor.
6. The Dietitian, with their manager, will plan CPD and identify training needs to meet contracted work and the cost will be incorporated into the pricing structure for the dietetic service.	6. There is evidence that the Dietitian and manager agree a programme which relates to the needs of the service in line with departmental CPD strategy.
7. The Dietitian identifies through evaluation whether ongoing objectives of CPD are met.	7. The Dietitian is able to identify and explain whether: • objectives have been met • practice has been enhanced • further development/education is required.

Table 7.2 British Dietetic Standard on continuing competence to practise[6]

A personal development plan has three main parts:

- What am I trying to do?
- How am I going to do it?
- This is what I need in order to do it.

A simple rule to remember when constructing learning objectives and personal development plans is to be SMART, i.e.:

Stretching and specific – the objectives should be challenging and focused
Measurable – how will success be measured?
Appropriate – do the personal objectives deal with issues that are important to both the individual and the organisation/team etc?
Realistic – are the objectives achievable (i.e. within resources available)?
Time-limited – are there time scales specified?

In identifying the personal objectives in the PDP, the following steps are helpful:

1. Begin by thinking in terms of:
   - MAINTAINING existing professional knowledge and skills
   - ENHANCING this knowledge and skill base
   - EXTENDING the current knowledge and skills.
2. Then consider the goals of the team and organisation, and see how the PDP fits in with these. This is important, as clinical governance links PDPs with organisation development plans – including, for example, practice development and locality plans for primary care.
3. Finally, consider whether certain requirements for professional development need to be satisfied (e.g. post-registration education and practice), how knowledge and skills have been developed in the past, and the preferred method of learning and studying (see CPD activities above).
4. To make the plan realistic and achievable, 6 objectives is an optimum number – no more than 10 should be identified.

Professional development is most likely to be of value when the learning:[8]

- builds on what is already known by the learner
- is driven by the learner's own identified needs
- has active participation
- uses resources known and easily available to the learner
- includes relevant, constructive and timely feedback
- has an element of self-assessment.

Key areas	Education and training needs	Possible activities	What I need to do to achieve this	Completed by (time scale)	How will I know I've succeeded? (Include a review date, e.g. 3 or 6 months)	Has this been achieved? Yes/No Comments – what I learnt from this
Objective one						
Objective two						
Objective three etc.						

Table 7.3 Personal development plan

The PDP can now be mapped out (Table 7.3). Separate maps can be charted for short-term goals (e.g. 1 year) and for longer-term goals (e.g. 3-5 years). The PDP is generally used in a one-to-one appraisal, a performance review process and mentoring.

There are also supporting processes for professional development. These include mentoring, peer review and clinical supervision. These processes, which are used by different health professionals, address different aspects of development in a confidential supporting environment, and can be conducted on an individual or team basis.

Mentoring:
A supportive nurturing relationship which provides inspiration and help by a mentor to a mentee to enhance the latter's skills and confidence.
Clinical supervision:
A formal process of professional support and learning which enables individual practitioners to develop knowledge and competence, assume responsibility for their own practice and enhance consumer protection and safety of care in complex clinical situations.[9]
Peer review:
An assessment of the quality of care provided by a clinical team with a view to improving patient care.

Professional self regulation

This process allows health professionals the opportunity to set their own standards of professional practice, conduct and discipline. To justify this freedom and maintain the trust of patients and their families, the professions are required to be accountable in an open manner for the standards they set and the way in which these are enforced. CPD is becoming one of the accepted methods of setting and monitoring standards relating to professional development.

The General Medical Council (GMC) is the UK regulatory body for doctors, and its function is to protect patients and maintain a register of doctors licensed to practice medicine. The Nursing and Midwifery Council (NMC) (the successor to the United Kingdom Central Council for Nursing, Midwifery and Health Visiting) serves a similar function for the nursing profession. The NMC requires nurses to maintain their professional registration through the process of PREP (post-registration education and practice).[10] If no evidence of continuous professional development is produced at the time of renewal, then the registration of the nurse lapses. Until recently no such mechanism was in place for doctors. However, the GMC is currently introducing a revalidation process for all doctors, who need to demonstrate that their knowledge is up-to-date in order to remain on the medical register.[11]

Regulation has been tightened up in another area. In 2002, the Council for Professions Supplementary to Medicine was replaced by a Health

Professions covered by the Health Professions Council:

- Art, drama, music and dance therapists
- Chiropodists
- Clinical scientists in health
- Dieticians
- Medical laboratory science officers
- Occupational therapists
- Paramedics
- Prosthetics and orthotists
- Physiotherapists
- Orthoptists
- Radiographers
- Speech and language therapists.

Professions' Council (HPC).[12] The new body has tighter controls on registration, and requires evidence from its members on fitness to practise, in order for them to remain on the register.

In addition to the changes to the individual professional regulatory bodies outlined above, a new body, the UK Council of Health Regulators, has been established to act as a forum in which common approaches across professions could be addressed (e.g. complaints against practitioners). The body has members from the GMC, NMC, HPC, the General Dental Council, the General Optical Council, the Royal Pharmaceutical Society, the General Osteopaths Council and the General Chiropractic Council.[13]

The picture is changing for health service managers too. The Institute of Healthcare Management requires all of its members to sign up to the IHM Management Code of Conduct, to have a baseline qualification and to undergo CPD in order to demonstrate 'fitness to practise'.[14]

Ultimately, the effectiveness of CPD as a process for clinical/professional or managerial development depends on the organisation's approach to creating a positive culture of learning. If it works well, then CPD is a useful mechanism for identifying under- or poor performance, through an appraisal or review system, and actions can be put in place to remedy the problems.

Table 7.4 Characteristics of poorly performing organisations[8]	
Individual	Poor performance (clinical and/or interpersonal care), low motivation
Organisation	Poor communication within clinical teams and managers, poor infrastructure, ineffective procedures for anticipating and handling management and clinical problems
Culture	Little sense of responsibility for patient care or staff/ colleagues' welfare. Education, research and professional development not valued
External relations	Little attempt to make professional contact outside of immediate sphere of work, unwillingness to discuss potential quality issues

It is important to be aware that organisations can also perform poorly. Although CPD is the building block of individual performance, other factors can influence the approach to learning. It is with this situation in mind that accreditation of organisations is becoming an important process to support the development of clinical governance.

Accreditation

There is an increasing trend to using external accreditation processes within the NHS. A number of organisations are entering the picture, including the medical Royal Colleges. In Scotland, this is being developed further by the National Standards Board and is mandatory. For the rest of the UK, external accreditation remains optional.

Table 7.5 The main components of accreditation	
Standards	These are predetermined, nationally set, easy to measure and consistent, and are updated regularly
Implementation	Examining the implementation and interpretation of the standards over a period of time (e.g. 1 year)
Measurement	A number of methodologies can be used, e.g. peer review or professional assessor, inspection of documents and site visits
Information	Including recommendations for future improvement (with or without an action plan) and the presentation of an award or grading.

Accreditation is a dynamic process that examines standards over a period of time and looks at different aspects – e.g. organisations (hospitals, primary care trusts), or specific services (e.g. a department of radiology, diabetes services across primary and secondary care, asthma care).

Examples of external accreditation schemes

Investors in people

This scheme sets a level of good practice for the training and development of staff to achieve business goals. This is not specific to health service organisations.

Investors in people give a planned approach to setting and communicating business goals, and developing staff to meet these goals. The result is that what staff can do and are motivated to do matches what the organisation requires them to do.

The investors in people standard also provides the basis for continuous improvement of both the organisation and its staff. The process requires a portfolio of evidence on 24 indicators to be submitted followed by an inspection by two assessors. Details are available from local Training and Enterprise Councils (TECs).

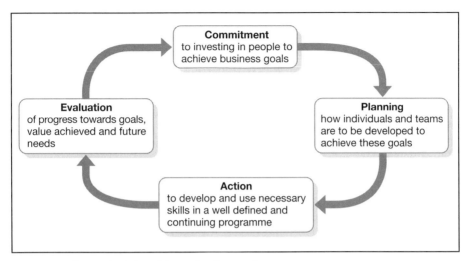

Figure 7.2 Four principles of investing in people

The four principles which underpin the process appear in Figure 7.2.

The charter mark

This is an award for public sector organisations, which requires continued submission of evidence every 3 years. Organisations have to show measurable and demonstrable improvements in the quality of service across a range of topics, and have plans for at least one innovative improvement to their quality of service. There is no on-site inspection.

ISO 9000 (formerly BS 5750)

This scheme focuses on sets of procedures to ensure accountability and systematic review of services provided by an organisation according to national standards. It is not specific to the health service. There must also be systems in place for feedback from users. An inspection is carried out. Details are available from local Training and Enterprise Councils (TECs).

RCGP quality practice award

This has been developed by the Royal College of General Practitioners, and the primary purpose is to promote and recognise good practice. Standards are set in 19 areas, largely in organisational aspects of the practice. The award is granted for 5 years.

RCGP team-based practice accreditation programme

This is another accreditation programme, again developed by the Royal College of General Practitioners, which is intended for quality improvement and practice development. This assesses two main areas; services to patients and the primary care team.

There is a danger that organisations and teams can become slaves to one of these quality initiatives. It is easy to become complacent once the achievement has been awarded, and to allow standards to slip.

Human resources and workforce planning

Having the appropriately trained staff in the right places at the right time to provide the care that is needed is essentially the purpose of workforce planning. The link between high quality service delivery and good

Table 7.6 Four pillars of good HR practice[15]

Pillar one – making the NHS a good employer

- Facilitative (including leadership) and involving management style – not hierarchical or controlling
- Better working conditions
- Model employment practices
- The ability to balance life inside and outside work
- Job security
- Lifelong learning
- Fair pay
- Staff involvement
- Good communications (three way communication – top/down, bottom/up and across)

Pillar two – the skills escalator

- Careers with a succession of stages, each with its own pay band and learning requirements
- Lifelong learning – allowing staff to constantly renew and extend skills and knowledge – 'moving up the escalator' through the support of the NHS University (see below)
- Roles and workload passed 'down the escalator' – giving greater job satisfaction
- Offering a wide variety of step-on and step-off points
- Effective workforce planning through workforce development confederations (see below)

Pillar three – improving staff morale

- Engaging staff in discussion about morale, including pay and conditions, pressures of workload, fear of litigation and increasing patient expectations

● Expressing publicly all that is good about the NHS

Pillar four – building people management skills

● All executives to appreciate HR issues
● Further development of the national HR management development programme, including a range of HR leadership development programmes from junior to board level.

Functions of WDCs[17]

WDCs:
● Take the lead on workforce planning for all health care disciplines, and help employers to improve workforce planning skills locally
● Take overall responsibility for developing the health care workforce, working with employers to develop and commission training programmes for all staff
● Catalyse the vision for the future health care workforce, helping employers to develop new ways of working (in conjunction with the workforce changing programme), challenging practice and promoting initiatives to improve staff retention
● Manage the education levy covering all the health care disciplines from three former budgets (the Non Medical Education and Training (NMET) budget, the Medical and Dental Education Levy (MADEL) and the Service Increment for Teaching (SIFT) budget)
● Negotiate and manage education contracts, working with local education and training providers
● Develop quality assurance programmes for health care education and training.

---

management of staff is the cornerstone of good employment practice. The document *HR in the NHS Plan*[15] sets out four pillars of good human resources practice:

● Making the NHS a model employer
● The skills escalator
● Improving staff morale
● Building people management skills.

Issues for consideration

Consider the four pillars of good HR strategy.

● Which areas have been implemented in your organisation?

- How successful has your organisation been in ensuring the involvement of the workforce in the planning and delivery of health care?

The process of workforce planning has undergone much change since the late 1990s, moving from a very central approach to a more locally sensitive method of planning the health service workforce. The process encompasses both long-term and short-term perspectives in the education and training of health professionals.

Following the Commons Health Select Committee's inquiry on the future of NHS staffing in 1999, and consultation on improving workforce planning in the NHS, local Workforce Development Confederations (WDCs) were established in 2001.[16]

The 24 WDCs spanning England have membership drawn from all the NHS bodies and local authority social service departments in the area they cover, the relevant postgraduate medical and dental deanery, education providers (universities, medical schools and colleges of further and higher education), representatives from the voluntary and independent sectors, the prison service and the Ministry of Defence (as appropriate). In addition to their core functions for the NHS, WDCs are also involved in workforce planning and training for social care organisations, prisons and the private and voluntary sectors.

Roles of the NHS university[18]

The NHS university:
- Develops a core curriculum (common learning programme) for all health professionals
- Acts as a signpost to existing training
- Provides a range of foundation, first-line and basic training programmes
- Provides quality assurance and accreditation for existing training
- Develops evaluation tools to measure how education improves patient care.

The NHS university

The NHS university (NHSU), established in 2003, is the biggest university in the world. Created to provide NHS staff with continuing access to high quality education and training, the NHSU is both a real 'bricks and mortar' institution and a virtual body. It plays an important role in ensuring that the learning and development needs of NHS staff are covered and are linked to the strategic direction of the NHS Plan.

Staff working in or for the NHS are nominally students of the NHSU. The intention is that all staff will begin their NHS career with the NHSU, either through induction or direct training. Then, personal development plans formulated by staff/students themselves will set a clear direction to which the university can respond by offering skills training, vocational training and education and academic development.

The NHSU works with WDCs and academic institutions; however, it does not replace the degree level courses for doctors, nurses and dentists which are still available at universities.

E-learning

Computer-based learning which provides access to training materials via web-based and networked technology. Training may be tailored to the individual's needs, and individuals are given performance support.

The NHSU is based on the principle of e-learning, with a central hub supported by local resource centres and facilities. The central hub draws on national strategies for human resources and lifelong learning, in partnership with WDCs, to produce innovative online learning packages and training and support programmes for NSFs, with guidance from NICE and CHAI.

Information management and technology

What is information, management and technology (IM&T)?

Information management is the provision of accurate, timely and (unless limited for security reasons) accessible information, when required, to support clinical and management decision making. This can be paper-based, electronic or verbal. The technology is the means by which the information is recorded and delivered.

The comprehensive quality improvement programme, which is one of the main components of clinical governance, is dependent on good information from a number of sources. These include:

- local clinical audit data
- national comparative data
- local care pathways, clinical guidelines and protocols (see Chapter 5)
- guidelines from the National Institute for Clinical Excellence (see Chapter 1)
- international research evidence (see Chapter 4).

The IM&T strategy objectives (1998-2005)[19]

- Lifelong electronic health records for every person in the country
- Round-the-clock on-line access to patient records and information about best clinical practice for all NHS clinicians
- Genuinely seamless care for patients from GPs, hospital and community services sharing information across the NHS information highway
- Fast and convenient public access to information and care via on-line services and telemedicine
- Effective use of NHS resources by providing managers with the information they need.

The government launched a national infrastructure development programme for information, management and technology in 1998, called *Information for Health,*[19] which set out a strategy for the NHS until 2005. The aims of the strategy are: to ensure that information is used to help patients receive the best possible care; for health professionals to have the information they need to provide that care; and to provide accurate information for managers to support local Health Improvement and Modernisation Programmes and the NHS Performance Assessment Framework. Further updates on the IM&T strategy have been produced; however, the targets remain largely the same.[20,21]
The key infrastructure developments are:

- Electronic patient records (EPR) and electronic health records (EHR)
- The NHS number – a unique number that identifies a patient using the NHS; every individual is given a number and keeps it all their life, and the same number is used whether the person uses GP or hospital services
- The NHS strategic tracing service – a service provided to NHS organisations to enable them to obtain an NHS number for individual patients
- NHSnet – a communications network designed to support electronic communications between NHS users quickly and securely; it is only accessible to the NHS

- The NHS information authority – a special health authority whose function is to lead the implementation of the Information for Health Strategy
- A national clinical information programme – a national initiative to co-ordinate and develop work on clinical information, including clinical record management, data quality, education and professional development, confidentiality issues and Read codes
- An NHS-wide clearing service – a national service for ensuring the quick and efficient transfer of the NHS minimum data sets and to support the production of nationally required statistics on NHS activity
- NHS Direct – a nationwide telephone service to the public, providing advice on health and health services
- Telemedicine/telecare – any health care related activity (including diagnosis, advice, treatment and monitoring) that involves a health professional and a patient (or two or more health professionals) who are separated in space (and possibly time) which is facilitated by the use of information and communication technology. Telemedicine is usually delivered in a hospital or surgery setting, whereas telecare is delivered in the patient's home.

Electronic patient records and health records

Electronic patient record (EPR)	This describes an episode of care provided mainly by one organisation (e.g. a period of time spent in hospital for a total hip replacement, or in a specialist unit or mental health NHS trust).
Electronic health record (EHR)	This describes the health care of a person from cradle to grave in all settings, including the outcomes of the periodic episodes of care held in the EPR.

The NHS has, for a long time, depended on paper-based clinical records. The IM&T strategy proposed the development of electronic records to facilitate the integration of care across different health sectors, to improve the accuracy of patient notes and to provide information for clinical audit, research and other quality assurance measures in an easily analysable form. Over time, the electronic record will replace the paper-based systems that are currently held separately. The success of these initiatives will depend on training all staff in accurate keyboard skills.

The Caldicott principles[22]

- Justify the purpose(s) for which information is required
- Don't use patient-identifiable information unless it is absolutely necessary
- Use the minimum necessary patient-identifiable information
- Access to such information should be on a strict 'need to know' basis
- All personnel with access should be aware of their responsibilities
- Understand and comply with the law.

The fact that valuable information in the NHS relates to individual patients and is generally gathered in confidence by health professionals needs to be safeguarded. This is applicable to electronic as well as to paper records. A review was undertaken by a committee chaired by Dame Fiona Caldicott concerning the uses made of patient-identifiable information for non-clinical purposes in order to determine the extent to which the flows of this type of information were justified and protected.[22]

A key component of the report is the establishment of Caldicott guardians to oversee access to patient-identifiable information, both within NHS organisations and at the Department of Health. The recommendation is that the guardian should be, in order of priority:

- an existing member of the board of the organisation
- a senior health professional
- an individual with a responsibility for promoting clinical governance within the organisation.

Typically the guardian is:

- in a strategic health authority, the Director of Public Health
- in an NHS trust, a board level clinician
- in a PCT, a board member with clinical governance responsibilities
- in each GP practice, a nominated lead person for confidentiality and security issues.

The national electronic library for health

The purpose of the National Electronic Library for Health (launched in 1999) is to provide easy access to the research papers and reviews on best current knowledge about health problems and their causes, prevention and treatment. It is a virtual library, bringing together the best national and international knowledge, based on technology used by the Internet.

The library has the following virtual 'floors', each of which has been developed in partnership with organisations that have expertise in the field:[23]

1. NHS Direct Online – this is the first section of the library to be developed and is dedicated to providing public information. It can be accessed through www.nhsdirect.nhs.uk
2. The know-how floor – this has been developed in partnership with the National Institute for Clinical Excellence and other organisations, and contains information such as the NICE guidelines, the National Service Frameworks, a separate care guidelines database and a care pathways database
3. The knowledge floor – this has been developed in partnership with the health care library community and contains information, amongst other things, on the British National Formulary, the British Library's electronic table of contents database (with the tables of contents of over 20,000 scientific journals and 16,000 conference proceedings published per year), Clinical Evidence (a database of clinical questions designed to help clinicians make evidence-based medical decisions) and the Cochrane Library
4. A reference section – this contains dictionaries, information on telemedicine, medicines and quality, and clinical governance.

The library has professional portals with clearly identifiable uni-professional entry points for various users including nurses, physiotherapists, occupational therapists, speech and language therapists, podiatrists, orthoptists, midwives, psychologists, dieticians and radiographers.

Like any library, the National Electronic Library for Health has two types of collections: a general collection and a series of special collections. The latter appears in the format of virtual branch libraries which contain information on specific conditions (such as coronary heart disease or cancers) and are maintained by experts in the appropriate fields who are supported by links with relevant stakeholder groups such as charities and patient organisations.

The NHSnet

The NHSnet is a secure national network developed exclusively for the NHS for conveying electronic information. In addition to being the medium for carrying patient information, it also serves an e-mail function and provides information on performance, good practice, health alerts and similar messages for those working in the NHS.

There are a number of services available on the NHSnet to NHS users, including:

- Electronic mail, to allow NHS users to send e-mails with attachments to recipients on the NHSnet and Internet
- An electronic data exchange (EDI) which enables electronic registration and items of service claims to be transferred between GP practices and PCTs. Similar links between hospitals enable the quick transfer of pathology and radiology results to GPs. Telemedicine services have been developed to allow health professionals in one location to access the advice and support of colleagues in another and, if appropriate, to enable discussions between professionals concerning patient consultations and treatments
- The NHSweb, which contains websites from a number of NHS organisations and has health databases and training support services for users connected to the NHSnet
- Internet access
- An on-line patient booking facility, which enables the direct booking of patients from general practice to outpatient appointments, and surgical operating lists (day cases and in-patients)
- Access to the National Electronic Library for Health.

The development of the NHS workforce and accurate information is as important in the functioning of clinical governance as the quality improvement activities discussed in earlier chapters. A theme that runs through all, however, is the involvement of patients, users and carers in the delivery of health care. This will be discussed in the next chapter.

References

1. Secretary of State for Health 1998 A first class service: quality in the new NHS. NHS Executive, London
2. NHS Executive 1999 Quality and performance – local delivery. In: The new NHS information pack. HMSO, London
3. The Institute of Health Services Management 1997 IHSM CPD support book [pilot scheme]. IHSM, London
4. Reay D G 1994 Understanding how people learn. Kogan Page, London
5. Knowles M 1975 Self-directed learning. Cambridge Books, New York
6. British Dietetic Association 1997 National professional standards for dietitians practising in healthcare. British Dietetic Association, Birmingham
7. Hutt M 1995 Continuing professional development: an action plan for you and the primary healthcare team; commissioned by North East Thames RHA. Anglia

Polytechnic University, Cambridge
8. Roland M, Holden J, Campbell S 1998 Quality assessment for general practice: supporting clinical governance in primary care groups. National Primary Care Research and Development Centre, University of Manchester, Manchester
9. Department of Health 1993 A vision for the future: report of the Chief Nursing Officer. HMSO, London
10. United Kingdom Central Council for Nursing, Midwifery and Health Visiting 1995 Standards for post-registration education and practice (PREP). UKCC, London
11. http://www.revalidationuk.info
12. Harris C 2002 Register rules. Health Service Journal 22nd August: 14-15
13. Department of Health 2002 The NHS plan: a plan for investment, a plan for reform. The Stationery Office, London
14. Foster R 2002 The realities of a code. Health Management 6(3): 23
15. Department of Health 2002 HR in the NHS plan. http://www.doh.gov.uk/hrinthenhs
16. Department of Health 2001 Investment and reform for NHS staff: taking forward the NHS Plan. The Stationery Office, London
17. http://www.doh.gov.uk/workdevcon/guidance.htm
18. Wyatt J 2002 Learning for all. Health Management 6 (7): 10-11
19. Secretary of State for Health 1998 Information for health. NHS Executive, London
20. Department of Health 2001 Building on the information core: implementing the NHS plan. The Stationery Office, London
21. Department of Health 2002 Delivering 21st century IT support for the NHS. The Stationery Office, London
22. NHS Executive 1997 Review of patient identifiable information: report of a committee chaired by Dame Fiona Caldicott. NHS Executive, London
23. NHS Information Authority 2001 National electronic library for health [information leaflet]. NHS Information Authority, London

8

The user perspective on the quality of care

How can we achieve the closer involvement of patients and the wider community?

> ... modern and dependable treatment ... must be delivered with ... a real understanding of patients' fears and worries.
> *A First Class Service*[1]

The earlier chapters have demonstrated that clinical governance is a complex concept. The disciplined and structured activities which will be necessary to achieve the required accountability frameworks and standards of excellence will touch on and influence many other existing tasks and systems. As we have seen, clinical audit activities, complaints, quality initiatives, formation and use of guidelines, and developing and using the evidence base for clinical and management roles are all influenced by the development of clinical governance.

This chapter argues that the service users' perspective must be an important part of all these activities and an integral thread in the discourse of clinical governance if we are to achieve the aims set out in *A First Class Service*. The Government sees the national survey of patient and user experience as being of crucial importance in disseminating information about the service user's perspective.

Unfortunately, experience indicates that although quite a considerable body of such information has already been built up, it has had limited impact on services and clinical behaviour. This is why the user's perspective needs to be at the heart of clinical governance and an integral part of all those activities cited above, which are the necessary foundations of clinical governance.

We may ask why the existing knowledge of service users' views has had little impact. In *Whose Standards?* Williamson[2] puts forward the view that some standards are 'intuitively' perceived as 'higher' or 'lower' than others, and explains why. The difference between professionals' and users' interests and power mediates perceived value. However, over time, 'professional ideology can accommodate new definitions of best interests' and thus, gradually, professionals may 'come to accept some consumerist standards for treatment and care'.

The picture of recent history (from the 1960s onwards) in the NHS represented in this seminal book is instructive. Time and time again the author recounts the struggles made by pressure groups representing patients to achieve acceptance of standards valued by users and their families. Frequently their efforts have met with resistance and they have taken years to achieve success. It is instructive to realise how many of those struggles were for standards of care that are now taken for granted and part of the received wisdom of good practice; for example, free parental access to children in hospital, or the presence of fathers during childbirth.

It is hoped that the implementation of clinical governance will provide an opportunity to build a better way of improving quality, but that can only be done if the service users' perspective is built into a range of activities and concepts, not least the notion of quality.

Quality in health care tends to be defined by clinicians in terms of clinical effectiveness, and by managers in terms of the range of efficiency measures that have been extensively developed through contracts and contract monitoring. However, quality is a complex concept, and depends significantly on the standpoint on the individual.

The complexity of quality

A case study

An 18-year-old woman suddenly started having fits. It became clear that these were going to be more than isolated or infrequent occurrences, so a referral for specialist assessment was made. There was a long wait for an initial appointment, partly due to the leave arrangements of relevant consultants. During this time the frequency and severity of the episodes increased, and although some diagnostic tests were arranged and medical staff had clear information about the episodes (following crisis A&E attendances) no treatment plan could be initiated until the consultant appointment.

Eventually, following the consultant appointment, a diagnosis of epilepsy was confirmed and anticonvulsant medication prescribed. Unfortunately, the required dosages on the prescription were unclear to the pharmacist, who sought the GP's advice. The GP was unfamiliar with the medication and sought clarification from the consultant. It proved difficult to establish contact with the consultant, and thus several more days passed before the young woman started taking the medication. Similar slowness in response and liaison with the GP meant that increasing the dosage because of limited response to the medication also took several days to agree and implement.

The family was worried about the young woman's emotional reactions to the diagnosis and were concerned that she needed help to ensure that her own behaviour and lifestyle should minimise risk and to come to terms with the diagnosis. At the time of diagnosis, no written material or counselling was offered to the young woman to help her to understand her condition, how it might affect her lifestyle, and how she might help herself. The family obtained a range of excellent publications produced by national voluntary agencies, and negotiated access to a nurse practitioner providing advice for children diagnosed with epilepsy.

This case study illustrates the complexity of quality, and how what constitutes quality may appear very different to service users and to clinicians. From the clinicians' standpoint, staff were looking at their service in terms of the diagnostic and assessment procedures and clinical treatment offered, and were concerned that these should be evidence-based. From the family's standpoint, the quality of the service offered was limited by poor advice and information, poor links between specialist and primary care, and poor channels of communication to enable patient, family, GP and specialist staff to work quickly and effectively together. An important point to note is that often what matters most to patients and carers is how the little things and processes are implemented – the actual times of appointments, repetition of investigations and the number of different health care professionals seen who seem to request the same information. The one issue where there might have been a consensus concerned waiting times, and on that score issues about arranging cover were possibly as important as managing demand and scarce resources.

Quality as a concept must embrace more than just the clinical effectiveness notions that are important to clinicians and the efficiency measures (time to first appointment, to assessment, etc.) that are important to managers.

How might implementing clinical governance ensure that the next patient in a similar position will receive a better quality service from the trust involved? *A First Class Service*[1] sets out four main components of clinical governance for trusts:

1. Clear accountability arrangements for the overall quality of clinical care, with designated responsibilities for boards, Chief Executives and clinicians, and regular reports to boards
2. Comprehensive programmes of quality improvement activities, including full participation in audit, evidence-based practice and professional development and training
3. Effective policies and practice to manage risk
4. Effective procedures to identify and manage poor performance.

We may conceive of clinical governance as a process of continuing critical scrutiny in relation to those four areas. However, as the case study indicates, continuing critical scrutiny should be applied to issues such as access, waiting times, ensuring adequate cover for clinicians, arrangements for access to clinical advice outside outpatient appointments, arrangements to ensure appropriate information and education for patients and families, and appropriate links with primary and social care where necessary. Will the mechanisms for implementing clinical governance ensure continuing critical scrutiny across the issues that concern service users, as well as clinicians and managers?

How do we know what quality means to service users?

People who use health services in the UK have been articulating their views and concerns for many years and, as NHS organisations have increasingly sought to involve and consult stakeholders, there are now are now many ways in which those views are expressed.

Williamson[2] has charted the development of consumer pressure groups, working at national level and addressing health service issues, since the 1960s. Service users are frequently closely involved with such groups, which usually have a clear focus on achieving improvements or change in specific areas of health care. Sometimes, over a period of years, the standards that such groups promote gradually become accepted into mainstream thinking about service quality.

There are many associations founded on the mutual concerns and interests of specific groups of service users and on providing self help and support. Organisations such as Diabetes UK, the British Epilepsy Association, the National Schizophrenia Fellowship, the National Childbirth Trust etc. provide a range of services and support to service users and their families. Close and frequent contact with service users can help to build a comprehensive understanding of what quality means to them, across both service delivery and clinical issues. Telephone helplines are not only very valuable to users; they are an important channel of communication and source of information about users' experience and concerns.

Some groups, such as Age Concern, MIND, etc., act on behalf of a broader range of service users and address many issues, although quality and standards in health care are usually significant. Groups may differ considerably in their willingness to address quality in clinical care and in their willingness to work collaboratively with health services and professionals. Concepts of quality and principles may differ, and involving service users is by no means without controversy. SANE and MIND, for example, have campaigned for quite different goals to improve services for people with mental health problems. Such differences may reflect a diversity of views amongst services users and responses to key issues such as autonomy and control, which are significant themes in users' ideas of quality.

Community Health Councils (CHCs) were established 'to represent the public interest in the local NHS'.[3] While CHCs varied considerably in their roles and local priorities, and while some commentators questioned their effectiveness,[3] many put considerable effort into facilitating the involvement of service users and local people and articulating their views on quality.

Advocacy services exist to help people who are unable to speak for themselves (often as a result of a disabling condition) to make their views known and to regain the power to make informed choices about services. Advocacy services may support people with many different problems, but commonly are provided to assist elderly people and those with physical disabilities, learning disabilities and mental health problems. While advocates will address whatever issues users raise, health care is usually a significant concern, and thus services may build an invaluable understanding of service users' concerns about quality in health care. Unfortunately, such information may not be used at a local level to help improve services.

Agencies commissioning health services increasingly sought to involve users in reviewing services, developing commissioning plans and strategies and, to a lesser degree, developing specifications and monitoring the quality of services. Reflecting the perspective of local people and the experience of patients in health service planning is now an explicit role for primary care organisations, perhaps reflecting the degree to which user involvement in commissioning is now regarded as good practice. At a national level, the arrangements for developing National Service Frameworks include mechanisms for involving service users; members of the National Institute for Clinical Excellence and the Commission for Health Improvement include patient representatives (and so will CHAI); and the experience of service users is to be surveyed (see Chapter 1).

The NHS Plan developed this trend further by expressing a move away from a system of care in which patients are outside of the system, towards a new model where the voices of patients, their carers and the public are heard at every level of the service, thereby acting as a lever for change and improvement.[4] In response to a discussion document, *Involving Patients and the Public in Healthcare,*[5] a number of mechanisms were proposed to improve public involvement:[6]

At an NHS organisational level, there are:

- Patients' Forums – every NHS trust and PCT in England has to set up an independent Patients' Forum which is a statutory body made up of patients and others from the local community. The Forum has powers to inspect all aspects of the work of trusts, including service delivery provided by general practice, NHS work carried out in the independent sector and wider health issues such as the development of local delivery plans. One member is elected to serve on the trust board.
- Patient Advice and Liaison Services (PALS) – PALS provide 'on-site' help to patients within NHS trusts and are employed by and responsible to trusts. Their role is to provide information to patients about health and health services locally, including voluntary organisations and support groups. PALS play a key role in resolving concerns and problems quickly before they become serious. They may put patients in touch with specialist independent advocacy services if they wish to complain formally, and act as an early warning system for trusts and Patients' Forums by highlighting gaps in service. PALS are monitored by Patients' Forums.
- Independent Complaints Advocacy Services (ICAS). The services operate from the community-based premises of the Commission for Patient and Public Involvement in Health (see below) and provide independent support to people who want to complain. ICAS complements existing advocacy services.
- Local Authority Overview and Scrutiny Committees (OSCs) – This is a mechanism whereby locally elected council representatives can scrutinize local health services, calling local NHS Chief Executives and other NHS managers to account.

Community Health Councils were abolished in 2003.

At the national level, the following structures operate:

- The Commission for Patient and Public Involvement in Health (CPPIH) –

this body is responsible for making appointments to Patients' Forums and complements existing patient organisations. It sets national standards, and provides training and monitoring of PALS, Patients' Forums and the Independent Complaints Advocacy Services (ICAS). At the community level, the CPPIH operates through local networks which facilitate the involvement of local groups, enabling them to provide feedback on health services development and provision. Local networks also commission the ICAS to act for patients, carers or families who need independent support in making a complaint.

Principles for empowering the public and patients[6]

- Effective – strengthening the voice of communities and patients
- Accessible – helping people to use health services locally
- Accountable – methods are clear and transparent
- Integrated – mirroring the structure of the NHS
- Independent – to allow scrutiny of health services
- Adaptable – using best practice locally and ensuring high quality.

The Expert Patient Programme – an example of patient empowerment[7]

The Expert Patient Programme aims to introduce self-management training programmes run by people with chronic diseases. The programme consists of a short, time-limited course which is delivered by trained volunteers living with a long-term medical condition, to enable others to gain confidence in managing their own condition (self-efficacy). The course focuses on shared experiences and deals with issues such as pain, fatigue and low self-esteem. Practical advice on fitness, exercise, symptom and fatigue management, nutrition, dealing with emotions, communication with family and health professionals, better use of medication, living wills and power of attorney form the course content. Outcomes of such courses have shown that physical deterioration is slowed, self-efficacy and psychological state improve, the use of health promoting techniques increases, the number of visits to the doctor decreases and communication with health care professionals improves.

What do we know about quality from the service user's point of view?

Given the diversity of user involvement activity described above, it is not surprising that there is a significant body of information on users' ideas of quality, albeit dispersed across many organisations and groups, and sometimes known as anecdote or narrative. These limitations may make it difficult to access information or reduce its credibility in the eyes of professionals. Nonetheless, some very clear themes emerge time and again across many different initiatives.

Some examples of the standards or issues which have emerged as important to particular groups of service users, are reproduced here.

Quality standards developed in consultation with users of a rehabilitation centre, as given to new service users

While you are at the centre, you are entitled to:

● privacy, respect and dignity
● be treated as a whole person; for all your needs to be addressed – physical, economic, educational
● full information about your diagnosis and treatment
● multidisciplinary assessment of your needs (involving community professionals as well as those from the rehabilitation centre)
● full involvement in this assessment
● co-ordinated planning of action to be taken to meet your needs
● full involvement in this planning
● help with thinking about your needs now and in the future, and for your definition of your needs to be central to this process
● access to an independent advocate should you wish it.

This is the service which has been purchased on your behalf; if you do not feel you have received this service, please contact...

Reproduced from *The Power to Change – Commissioning Health and Social Services with Disabled People*[8]

Standards for health care services expressed by people with recurrent and chronic pain, and women with HIV, in a research study exploring patients' charters

Most important for people with pain is to be listened to, pain acknowledged, and not dismissed as a failure, and then:
● support and advice on pain management within weeks of the pain developing
● referral to specialist pain management programmes within 2 years of pain developing
● regular review of their condition – in case a new drug or treatment is available
● support and advice for carers and family
● multidisciplinary assessment and choice of treatments, including non-conventional therapies available in primary care
● practical help in coping with other aspects of life affected by the condition – income, childcare, mobility.

Most important for women with HIV is:
- confidentiality of information and acknowledgement that it is up to them to choose who to inform
- respect for autonomy and the right to make own decisions about their life, such as pregnancy
- support and counselling
- regular review and monitoring by a specialist centre
- care shared between the GP and hospital
- joint assessment and choice of treatments, including non-conventional therapies, available in primary care
- support and advice for carers and family
- practical help in coping with other aspects of life affected by the condition – income, childcare, housing.

Reproduced from *Working with Users – Beyond the Patients Charter*[9]

The NHS Executive produced a strategy for enhancing patient involvement in service development.[10] It stated that working collaboratively in patient partnership should have four overall aims.

At the level of individual patient care:
- to promote user involvement in their own care, as active partners with professionals
- to enable patient to become informed about their treatment and care and to make informed decisions and choices about it if they wish.

At the level of overall service development:
- to contribute to the quality of health services by making them more responsive to the needs and preferences of users
- to ensure that users have the knowledge, skills and support to enable them to influence NHS service policy (see Chapter 4 on critical appraisal).

Issues for consideration

Consider the initiatives within your organisation that have involved patient views and perspectives.

- What areas of service delivery have changed as a result of this process?

Service users' views on developing primary care were also sought as part of discussions on the future of primary care in 1996, and are summarised from *Primary Care: The Future*:[11]

- People wish to become more actively involved in care, making informed choices about the treatment options available to them and about the way services should be developed
- A continuing personal link with members of the primary health care team can facilitate this active involvement
- Information about the range and quality of health services, treatments and health promotion should be widely available in surgeries and pharmacies
- Better clinical information should be available to people in accessible forms
- Advocacy should be available to people who need special help in accessing services
- The personal relationship between patient and GP is a cornerstone of primary health care.

Methods of involving patients in primary care[12]

- Questionnaires, surveys and patient satisfaction audits
- Focus groups (targeting specific issues)
- Patient participation groups (ongoing, wider remits)
- Consultation on various plans (e.g. practice development plans)
- Newsletters.

Studies and initiatives such as these indicate particular quality issues for specific groups of people. However, the common themes that tend to emerge across many different initiatives may indicate aspects of quality that need to be taken on board by all services. This was highlighted in many of the recommendations made by the public inquiry into failures in the performance of surgeons involved in heart surgery on children at Bristol Royal Infirmary between 1984 and 1995.[13]

Key recommendations made in the Bristol Royal Infirmary Inquiry[13]

- Involve patients/parents in decisions
- Keep patients/parents informed of progress
- Improve communication with patients/parents
- Provide parents with counselling and support if needed
- Obtain informed consent for all procedures and processes
- Elicit the views of patients/parents and listen to their opinions
- Be open and candid when adverse events occur.

Involving patients is a central theme of the NHS Plan and, as noted above, a number of principles or themes have been developed for successful patient and public involvement.

These common themes are briefly discussed below.

Aspects of quality

Information

In the case discussed above, the lack of helpful information was experienced as a serious limitation on the quality of care. People want information about their condition, both short-term and long-term; about how they could or should modify their lifestyle as a result of the condition; about treatments, treatment choices, advantages and disadvantages of treatments (including 'alternative' treatments, dietary regimes etc.); and about services available. Families and carers also have a similar range of information needs.

Adequate and helpful information can be crucial in assisting people in adjusting to their condition, in full understanding of and compliance with treatment, and in securing the necessary practical and emotional support from carers. There is also some evidence to suggest that comprehensive information prior to clinical intervention can improve outcome.[2]

For many clinicians, however, providing information may present dilemmas. Lack of time is the most obvious constraint, although ensuring appropriate written information or working with relevant patients' organisations are ways of addressing the difficulty. Clinicians may also be worried that information can raise anxiety. Initiatives to explore what information people want and need on admission to acute psychiatric care have shown that nurses and other practitioners may feel concerned about information increasing people's worries, while the people themselves clearly want more information than they may be given. They often feel that information giving should be gradual, responding to the changing situation, rather than too much at once. The complexities of what an individual may need or be able to take in and understand, or may find alarming, at any one time, imply a need for sufficient time and subtle judgement on the part of clinicians.

Choice

Information is essential for choice and informed consent. People may wish to exercise choice:

- about whether or not to have treatment
- about different types of treatment

- about where (which hospital or centre) and from whom (which clinician, or care manager/key worker) to receive treatment
- about the setting for treatment (home, day care, in-patient)
- about what is the important problem to tackle first (e.g. people with mental health problems may prioritise their urgent accommodation or money problems rather than psychological symptoms).

Recent government policies on publishing information about the performance of hospitals and units may, over time, increase the opportunity for choice.

Choice also implies that patients need to be competent to make decisions about treatments, and in some cases clinicians may be faced with difficult situations if a patient's choice to take or refuse care may endanger his or her life (see Chapter 10).

Quality of life and practical aspects of living

Clinicians and practitioners understandably prioritise improving medical conditions and symptom relief. For many patients, however, particularly those with conditions which are long term or which may have disabling effects, the quality of life may be paramount. The capacity to communicate, go out, be involved in social events, follow stimulating interests and pursuits, participate in meaningful activity, continue to work, maintain personal and sexual relationships, sleep, think clearly, and maintain self-esteem and self-confidence, all contribute to quality of life. All may be diminished by illness or by treatments; conversely, some interventions may positively improve quality of life. For some people these issues will be very important in terms of choices about health care and other forms of care and support. Here, new treatments that potentially improve the quality of life (e.g. a new drug for the treatment of rheumatoid arthritis) but cause funding problems for purchasers often raise ethical issues around who has access to health care.

Tools to empower patients[14]

- recognise patients' expertise, values and preferences
- offer informed choice, not passive consent
- training in shared decision making
- evidence-based decision aids for patients
- public education on interpreting clinical evidence
- patient access to electronic health records
- surveys of patients' experience to prioritise quality improvements
- openness and empathy with patients/parents after medical errors have occurred
- public access to comparative data on quality and outcomes.

Co-ordinated care

Increasingly, comprehensive care for an individual may involve a range of health care professionals, sometimes from a variety of organisations, and also practitioners from social services and voluntary sector agencies. Ensuring that care is co-ordinated and continuous becomes a critically important function, and key worker systems and care planning processes (such as the Care Programme Approach for mental health services, and Care Management for community care) are designed to achieve this. Information on service users' views indicates that co-ordinated care is a high priority and a major quality concern.

Control and decision-making

Being an active partner in making decisions about health care, and being to a greater or lesser degree in control of one's own health care, are major concerns for many service users. Self administration of medication or analgesia, patient-held records, self-assessment questionnaires (e.g. the 'Meeting Your Needs' form for people with mental health problems developed by Nottingham Advocacy Project[15]) are all helpful ways in which service users can exercise some self management, and share decision making. Where a service user's capacity to make decisions may be diminished in certain situations, they may be able to express their preferences beforehand. 'Living wills', in which people state their wishes regarding treatment in the case of terminal illness and imminent death, are probably the best known examples (see Chapter 10). For people with mental illness, crisis plans may be agreed between service users and practitioners in advance of situations in which their ability to decide is impaired.

Respect

The term 'respect' is mentioned frequently in service users' narratives, in declarations of rights (e.g. Declaration of Rights of People with Cancer) or user-initiated charters, and in many surveys and studies of users' views. It also figures significantly in complaints about staff attitudes and behaviour, and has thus become an important part of satisfaction surveys – usually as questions regarding courtesy. Respect as an aspect of quality may be defined in many ways, but is probably most frequently expressed in terms of being listened to and understood. Privacy and confidentiality may also be important aspects of respect. Essentially, respect means being treated as 'competent and valued adults'.[2]

The dilemma of diversity

While information, respect and co-ordinated care are probably important to all service users, some of the other aspects of quality will have a variety of meanings and weight, depending upon the individual. Individuals have different approaches to illness, and different ways of managing themselves and the stress of illness. Thus, people may have very different preferences about the amount and type of information they require, and the degree to which they wish to exercise choice and control.

This may present a real dilemma for clinicians. Clinical effectiveness and other quality initiatives use guidelines and uniform standards to achieve consistent good practice. Yet some of the aspects of quality that are most important to service users may not easily lend themselves to such practice. However, many people can identify their preferred coping strategies if invited to do so. This suggests that one aspect of quality in the dialogue between practitioners and service users may be the degree to which these preferences are openly recognised and influence different approaches to self-management and control.

Towards a broader concept of quality – and putting it into practice

Most clinicians and managers want to do a good job well; they demonstrate a commitment to quality. However, that commitment needs to be expanded; it should be a commitment to taking on board and putting into practice a concept of quality that incorporates the perspective and priorities of service users, as well as those of practitioners and managers. This is not easy to do; if it were, there might have been more progress in improving services in line with service users' concerns.

However, there are some methods and simple principles which may help us to root or embed a broader concept of quality into practice.

Care pathways

The care pathway process is designed to:

- track each stage of a service user's 'pathway' through care
- involve all professionals (and possibly other staff) who might be providing part of a service along that pathway
- develop a protocol for the best possible shape of the pathway and service delivery
- build in an audit of practice against the protocol that has been developed.

Service users participate in the process, clarifying both discontinuities along the pathway and their quality concerns. The involvement of all staff involved allows a much clearer picture of the stages of care, and different workers' contributions to that care. The pathway sets standards for what ought to happen and what ought to be achieved at each stage of care.

In terms of earlier discussion of quality, this is a tool that could be very helpful in bringing together clinicians', managers', and service users' perspectives of quality. It also could be very helpful in improving co-ordination of care, which is known to be a major aspect of quality for service users. Further details on care pathways appear in Chapter 5.

Client-focused or patient-defined outcomes

It is clear that the issues that mean quality in services to the users are not necessarily the same as those that are important to clinicians and managers. We can work with service users to capture those concerns, asking them to specify their own desired outcomes, and we can then build those outcomes into audit and monitoring activity[16] (see also Chapter 9).

On a practical basis it is sometimes easier to proceed down this track, working with groups of people using specific services. The existence of a relevant service users' organisation or group may provide help in reaching service users and structuring discussions from which more precise questions can be framed and outcomes drafted. It may also be important to recognise the differences between groups of people using services; desired outcomes for young women in the 20-30 years age group may well be different to those for Asian men in the 40 years plus age group, even if they are using the same service.

For individual service users, self-assessment formats or working with practitioners to set goals for care may also be important. These could be more routinely incorporated in practice, particularly for service users with long-term or disabling conditions or those that have a significant impact on ordinary life.

Service users' involvement in clinical and service audit

Service users can be effectively involved in all stages of the audit cycle, through selecting and prioritising topics, setting standards and criteria, monitoring treatment and care, disseminating findings and implementing change. The Department of Health has encouraged clinical audit committees to explore ways of incorporating the service users' perspective in audit, and in 1995 national surveys revealed that 20% and 24% of trust audit committees and Medical Audit Advisory Groups respectively, had already recruited, or intended to recruit, patient members.[17]

The College of Health, which works to represent the interests of patients and promote patient-centred care, gives examples[11] of a number of audit initiatives in which service users have participated. These include:

- a project to audit treatment of thyrotoxicosis at the interface between primary and secondary care, in which an individual patient was involved in all stages of the project
- an audit of a breast cancer service in which both professionals and service users were involved in setting service standards
- service user involvement in a range of activities to develop and test an audit system for a mental health service.

An audit project of a wheelchair service[18] provides an interesting reflection on some of the issues raised here concerning outcomes and audit, and some different methods and approaches. A local user group helped to identify seven distinct sub-groups of users with different needs and requirements of the wheelchair service. The group then identified assessment criteria or outcomes that were important to all users and carers, and criteria specific to sub-groups of users. Some further criteria to assess empathy, understanding and responsiveness of the service were developed, and all criteria were incorporated into a questionnaire agreed by users and professionals. The questionnaire allowed respondents to rate the importance of individual criteria as well as the performance of the service. Results were thus brought together in a matrix showing both degree of importance to service users of specific criteria and satisfaction with service, which was helpful in indicating necessary management action.

This study is interesting in the methods used to define user-focused outcomes that recognised the differences between different service users. It also built up criteria that could be used sytematically to measure aspects of 'empathy' which, given our earlier discussion of the importance of 'respect', is valuable.

Clinical governance as a process of continuing critical scrutiny

As stated at the beginning of this chapter, we may conceptualise clinical governance as a process of continuing critical scrutiny in relation to the quality of services. If that scrutiny is to result in services that service users experience as high quality, then the process of scrutiny must cover a wide range of service issues and not just focus on professional judgement.

Our discussion of the service users' perspective on quality indicates that clinical governance arrangements should incorporate:

- careful scrutiny of the organisation's structures for improving quality, to ensure that wherever possible service users are involved
- careful scrutiny of the organisation's programmes and initiatives to improve quality, to ensure that wherever possible, the methodologies adopted facilitate the identification and promotion of service users' perspectives on quality
- careful scrutiny of the information and advice given to service users and their families at each point on the care pathway, involving users and families to ascertain what information is needed and how to give it
- careful scrutiny of the role and importance of self-management in any particular condition, and requirements for user education and information
- careful scrutiny of the organisation of service delivery, including all parts of the care package and essential links with all practitioners, from whichever agency.

References

1. NHS Executive 1998 A first class service: quality in the new NHS. Department of Health, London
2. Williamson C 1992 Whose standards. Open University Press, Buckingham
3. Dabbs C 1999 Sold a pup: community health councils. Health Service Journal 20 May
4. Department of Health 2000 The NHS plan: a plan for investment, a plan for reform. The Stationery Office, London
5. Department of Health 2001 Involving patients and the public in healthcare: a discussion document. http://www.doh.gov.uk/involvingpatients
6. Department of Health 2001 Involving patients and the public in healthcare: response to the listening exercise. http://www.doh.gov.uk/involvingpatients
7. http://www.doh.gov.uk
8. Morris J 1995 The power to change: commissioning health and social services with disabled people. The Prince of Wales Advisory Group on Disability and The King's Fund, London
9. Hogg C 1994 Beyond the patients charter: working with users. Health Rights Ltd, London
10. NHS Executive 1996 Patient partnership: building a collaborative strategy. NHS Executive, London
11. NHS Executive 1996 Primary care: the future. HMSO, London
12. NHS Executive 1997 Primary healthcare teams: involving patients, examples of good practice. NHS Executive, London
13. Bristol Royal Infirmary Inquiry 2001 Learning from Bristol: the report of the public inquiry into children's heart surgery at the Bristol Royal Infirmary 1984-1995. The Stationery Office, London http://www.bristol-inquiry.org.uk
14. Coulter A 2002 After Bristol: putting patients at the centre. British Medical

Journal 324: 648-651
15. Nottingham Advocacy Group. Meeting your needs. Nottingham Advocacy Group, Nottingham
16. Kelson M 1999 Patient defined outcomes. College of Health, London
17. Kelson M 1998 Promoting patient involvement in clinical audit. College of Health, London
18. Dunleavy P, Farmer P 1996 Service quality audit: involving users and carers in the community. CCMP 4(5)

9

Evidence-based management

The previous chapters have discussed in detail the skills and developments required of clinicians to deliver evidence-based clinical care. This emphasis is appropriate with the establishment of clinical governance. However, there must also be a spotlight on the effectiveness of management processes within the Health Service for clinical governance to work. This is particularly pertinent because there have been examples in the past of poorly considered management decisions, such as the implementation of resource management or investment in new IT processes that have failed, leading to patchy uptake or a huge waste of money. It is important, therefore, to take a systematic and scientific approach in this area.

Approaches to evidence-based management[1]

- There should be a culture of finding, appraising and using research-based knowledge for all staff (including managers)
- All staff should have practical skills in appraising the evidence
- Information should be available in an easily accessible form, ideally using a computer
- An emphasis (particularly on managers) to ask, what is the evidence for this proposal or decision?

The essential components of an evidence-based service as identified by Muir Gray[1] are:

- Organisations that have the capability to generate and the flexibility to incorporate the research evidence
- Individuals and teams who are able to find, appraise and apply the research to routine clinical practice.

A third aspect can be added, and that is the monitoring of the outcomes of the application of the research evidence and changing clinical practice as appropriate (i.e. whether patients get better and if lessons are learnt through the process).

The key to supporting these processes is how effectively the managers within NHS organisations do their work, and whether their decisions are evidence based.

The promotion of evidence-based decision making must be encouraged from the Chief Executive downwards throughout the managerial as well as the clinical staff.

Effective managers

The NHS has been experiencing major change since the early 1990s, and this looks set to continue in the future. This, not surprisingly, is accompanied by role confusion, uncertainty and anxiety which is felt particularly by managers who are required to implement these changes smoothly, often against some resistance within their organisations. The importance of demonstrating effective evidence-based management has never been more apparent.

There is no doubt that effective managers are needed in organisations to ensure their smooth functioning and to ensure that services are provided.

Why organisations need managers[2]

- To ensure the organisation serves its basic purpose, i.e. the efficient production of goods or services
- To design and maintain the stability of the operations of the organisation
- To take charge of strategy making and adapt the organisation in a controlled way to changes in its environment
- To ensure the organisation serves the ends of the people who control it
- To serve as a key informational link between the organisation and the environment
- As formal authority to operate the organisation's status system.

A specific type of role is required for this to occur. A starting point could be an examination of the kinds of skills and attributes managers need in order to steer such a course.

Katz[3] identified three basic skills on which effective management depends (Table 9.1).

Table 9.1 Basic skills on which effective management depends[3]

Technical competence	The specialist knowledge, methods and skills applied to discrete tasks (e.g. budget setting, IT, decision making, clinical knowledge etc.)
Human and social skills	Interpersonal relationships and the exercise of judgement (i.e. motivating, selecting, developing other team members, persuasion and negotiation, enabling and empowering and other aspects of effective use of human resources)
Conceptual	The ability to see things as a whole, how one part affects another, and decision-making skills
A fourth skill was later added:	
Political	The use of both personal power and formal power/authority, including the interpretation of group behaviours, building consensus, positive influencing and managing conflict informally.

In terms of managerial activities, Kotter[3] identified two main areas:

- Agenda setting – this is a set of items or agendas which involve objectives, plans, strategies, ideas, priorities and decisions to be made in order to achieve desired end results
- Network building – meeting with people within and outside the organisation in order to assist in the successful achievement of agenda items.

Within this, there are the 10 essential roles of a manager's job as identified by Mintzberg:[2]

Table 9.2 Essential roles of a manager's job[2]

The interpersonal roles (leading)

Relations with other people arising from the manager's status and authority

1. Figurehead	Basic role, the manager represents the organisation in ceremonial activities (particularly pertinent to the Chief Executive), e.g. signing of documents, and being available for people who insist on access to the 'top'
2. Leader	A significant role, responsibility for staffing, motivation and guidance of others in the organisation
3. Liaison	Relationships with others outside the organisation

The informational roles (administrating)

Relates to sources and communication of information arising from the manager's interpersonal roles

4. Monitor	The seeking and the receiving of information from internal or external sources
5. Disseminator	The circulation of information within and outside of the organisation
6. Spokesperson	The formal authority for the transmission of information to people outside of the organisation, e.g. the public and other agencies

The decisional roles (fixing)

Relates to the making of strategic organisational decisions

7. Entrepreneur	The initiation and planning of change
8. Disturbance handler	Reaction to unpredictable events
9. Resource allocator	The allocation of resources to specific areas, e.g. time, money, staff and materials
10. Negotiator	The negotiation of contracts or service level agreements

The overriding managerial role is decision making. Managers need to consider other aspects of their job that may or may not facilitate the way they perform. Stewart[4] identified three main choices for the manager.

Table 9.3 Choices for the manager[4]

Demands of the job

What the manager *has* to do, including performance and behavioural demands:
- boss-imposed
- peer-imposed
- externally-imposed
- system-imposed
- subordinate-imposed
- self-imposed

Constraints placed on job holder by the job

Internal or external factors that impose limits on what the manager can do:
- resource limitations
- legal regulations
- union agreements

- technological limitations
- physical location of the manager and his/her unit
- organisational policies and procedures
- people's attitudes and expectations

Choices available to the job holder

The activities that the manager is free to do:
- what work is done
- how the work is done
- when the work is done
- what new initiatives might be developed

The Institute of Healthcare Management encapsulated these roles and requirements in their statement of primary values (1999).[5] This has now been developed as the code of conduct for NHS managers (see Chapter 10).

The Institute of Health Services Management (Institute of Healthcare Management from October 1999) statement of primary values[5]

This is a framework for decision making and action. In making decisions and taking actions, managers will:

For individuals
- respect the dignity of every individual
- respect and welcome diversity amongst patients, colleagues and the public
- listen to the views of others
- respect confidentiality of all patients and colleagues
- respect the professional standards to which colleagues owe allegiance

For the organisation
- use resources responsibly
- strive for accessible and effective health care according to need
- use processes which are open
- promote a climate in which patients, colleagues and the public can register concerns and where discussion is encouraged and valued
- provide equality of opportunity for personal development
- communicate with integrity, balance and clarity

On a personal level
- take personal responsibility
- be sensitive to the consequences for others of their actions
- ensure that their own skills, knowledge and experience are continually developed.

Issues for consideration

- If you have any management function in your current situation, consider the 10 roles of a manager as identified by Mintzberg and compare these with your job. Which are relevant and which are not?
- If your role is a clinical role only, how many of the main choices of a manager, as identified by Stewart, are relevant to you?

Although the specific jobs of managers differ widely, the characteristics discussed above apply in most managerial situations. On careful examination, some of the characteristics can even be applicable to the one-to-one clinical consultation – for example, the assessment is carried out using information obtained from either inside or outside the organisation as well as using specific skills and knowledge, the allocation of resources (i.e. treatment) needs to be decided on, and there may need to be liaison with other agencies (e.g. social services etc.).

One of the areas where the effective use of the evidence is beginning to be utilised is in the process of commissioning health care and monitoring these outcomes.

Evidence-based commissioning

The separation of the purchasers or commissioners of health care from the providers in the NHS allows the former to determine how best to use finite resources for patient groupings (e.g. children or older people), specific conditions (e.g. diabetes) or particular interventions (e.g. total hip replacements or endoscopies). Managers need to use the research evidence to support their commissioning decisions in order to justify the pattern of spending to the public and the tax payer. The process of evidence-based commissioning begins with an assessment of the needs of the population for which the care is to be provided.

Evidence-based needs assessment

Needs assessment is a method of quantifying the needs of a defined population which can be described in health terms (health care needs) or can include the wider social and environmental determinants of health, such as housing, education, lifestyle and employment and other sociological and economic factors.

What is needs assessment?

Needs assessment is:[6]
The systematic approach to ensuring the health service uses its resources to improve the health of the population in the most efficient way.

Health care needs can be defined as:[6]
People who benefit from health care, e.g. health promotion, disease prevention, medical and nursing treatment, rehabilitation and palliative care. This is what health care professionals provide; however, patients may have a different perspective of their needs (such as employment, a secure job, better housing and transport etc.).

Health needs:[6]
This area includes wider influences on health such as environmental factors, lifestyle, genetic makeup and health promoting/disease prevention activities.

The aim of needs assessment in the NHS is to provide the basis for ensuring the effective allocation of finite resources, which can be used to deliver the best value health care to patients. In reality, the process tends to be a balance between need, demand and supply.

- 'Need' is the capacity of people to benefit from an effective intervention, e.g. smoking cessation, dietary and alcohol advice and other lifestyle factors in the management of coronary heart disease. This need may not necessarily present to services.
- 'Demand' is what people ask for, and it can be generated by the media raising public expectations, the patient's own characteristics, or by supply, such as the variation in access to services (e.g. waiting times for elective surgery) (see Chapter 8 – involving users).
- 'Supply' is the actual health care that is provided by health services for a population. The pattern of health care provision has depended on historical interests of health professionals, the amount of funding available and the latest priorities of politicians. Supply does not necessarily relate to actual needs.

One of the main problems encountered in a needs assessment exercise is setting the scale and scope of the subject identified, particularly as there is usually a limited period of time and finite resources that can be devoted to this activity. Assessing needs tends to generate much discussion around access to care, and highlights current local problems; a strong handle should be kept to maintain the original course. Other common problems are:

- Data – too much or too little relating to the area studied, or data placed in many different locations or systems

- Which approaches to take or methods to use
- Loss of direction (usually halfway through the exercise)
- How is the need defined? Or is it looking at demand?
- Who defines the need or priorities?
- Raising expectations – beware 'unearthing' needs which may not be met.

This situation raises the question, what is the evidence for this proposal and how does this sit in the national and local policy framework? A needs assessment should be triggered by the importance of an identified health problem – how frequently it occurs, the impact on services or the cost etc. – or a critical incident such as a mentally ill patient discharged too early from hospital who then commits suicide. The subject of a needs assessment should be within the context of national or locally agreed priorities. In addition, with the increasing emphasis on evidence-based care, needs assessment can be used to examine the effectiveness of a new treatment and the effect of the research findings on the burden of disease.

Commissioning health care

Using the information obtained from a robust needs assessment, it is possible to accomplish the main evidence-based tasks[1] of allocation of resources, managing innovation and controlling costs.

The allocation of resources among and within disease management systems

Disease management systems are the services and interventions that are designed to improve the health of people who have a particular disease (e.g. asthma or diabetes) or a group of diseases (such as coronary heart disease). Historically, the NHS was dominated by broad distinctions between primary and secondary care or between hospital and community care due to discrete funding mechanisms. Reallocation of resources was therefore done on the basis of contracts for particular patient groups – outpatients, day cases, mental health, specific secondary care services such as gynaecology, orthopaedics etc. With the introduction of unified PCG budgets and the IM&T strategy developing the information base for packages of care (and the use of care pathways), these barriers are slowly being broken down. However, there is still a long way to go before such a process is commonplace.

Managing innovation

A purchaser is constantly faced with managing the introduction of innovation. The challenges are ensuring that innovations:

- that do more good than harm and are affordable are introduced at a particular standard of quality (i.e. promoting innovation)
- that do more harm than good are not introduced (i.e. preventing the start of this course of action)
- of unknown effect are investigated under controlled conditions (i.e. through trials)
- are reviewed regularly to monitor the effective use of resources.

The function of the National Institute for Clinical Excellence is to provide sound evidence for these processes in order to support both purchasers and clinicians (see Chapter 1). However, the harder challenge is trying to change established professional practice, rather than the introduction of a new drug.

Controlling increases in health care costs without affecting the health care of the population

Increasing health care costs can be due to ineffective methods of providing health care, such as the carrying out of procedures as an in-patient rather than a day case (e.g. cataract surgery). Here, pathways of care can help in identifying inefficiencies whilst at the same time safeguarding or even improving the standard of care provided (see Chapter 5).

> ### What is commissioning?
>
> A definition of commissioning is 'the process by which health needs of a population are defined and appropriate services purchased and evaluated in order to ensure maximum health gain'.[7] This process involves a complicated set of activities including 'assessment of need, the appraisal of options to meet the need, the evaluation of effectiveness of interventions and the prioritisation of competing needs for services, as a necessary preliminary to decisions about buying health care'.[8]

The process of commissioning generally follows these steps:[7]

- Assessing health needs of the population
- Audit of current service provision
- Developing a strategy with other partners
- Determining priorities according to national and local imperatives
- Evaluation – determining the scope and process of evaluation
- Submission of the commissioning plan
- Negotiation of service level agreements (contracts).

Sometimes not all the steps are followed; however, one of the key activities of the process is the development of a strategy for the service to be commissioned. Again, the evidence base plays an important role in order to justify the decision on the allocation of resources. A strategy is generally developed in the following way[7] and the method used is similar to that for achieving a change in behaviour (see Chapter 3):

● Identifying a rationale for the service generally (incidence, prevalence) – i.e. the needs assessment
● Identifying a rationale for the service on a local, regional and national level – i.e. which are the priorities?
● Describing of the service to be provided
● Reviewing national guidance, targets, indicators, clinical effectiveness etc.
● Agreeing a statement of principles and values underpinning the strategy and overview of the quality standards expected
● Stating the aims and objectives of the strategy, local targets and time scale for achievement
● Listing of key stakeholders involved in the strategy
● Providing a glossary and key references.

Evidence-based initiatives

The processes described above are used to a greater or lesser extent every year in the commissioning cycle between PCTs and other trusts. Increasingly the evidence is being examined to test assumptions about commissioning habits. For example, Johnstone and Zolese[9] carried out a systematic review of all randomised controlled trials comparing planned short stay versus long hospital stay or standard care for people with serious mental illness. They found that planned short hospital stays seemed to be as effective as long hospital stays for a number of outcomes, including readmission rates, losses to follow-up and timely discharge. Griffin[10] found in his meta-analysis that structured call and recall systems in general practice for patients with diabetes were as effective as outpatient hospital care. These findings have implications for future patterns of commissioning; however, although both papers conducted extensive searches for suitable trials to study, there were in fact very few that could be used to assess the criteria upon which the reviews were based. Clearly more research needs to be done to support evidence-based commissioning, as problems do occur.

The supraregional services advisory group (SRSAG) designated the Bristol Royal Infirmary (BRI) as one of nine centres for paediatric cardiac surgery in 1984, although it had only performed three such operations that year. The case in terms of a critical mass of work necessary to be achieved for such designation was very weak; however, it was an important geographical location. The SRSAG had hoped that, with designation and support from the Royal Colleges, referrals would increase and outcomes would improve. However, London hospitals continued to run clinics in the south-west, and patients continued to be referred to them. In addition, in 1986 the Welsh Office agreed in principle to set up a paediatric cardiac unit in Cardiff. The SRSAG monitored the number of cases going to the BRI, which failed to increase. Furthermore, the outcomes were not assessed. The Welsh Office at the highest level was aware of undercurrents of dissatisfaction with the work at BRI; however, no action was taken.[11]

In the case of the Bristol Royal Infirmary, the evidence for basing one of the regional paediatric cardiac surgery centres there was not robust. However, there have been a number of projects that have attempted to improve the implementation of evidence-based clinical care in a variety of settings.

Getting research into purchasing and practice (GRiPP)

This project, which was initiated by Oxford Regional Health Authority in 1993,[12] involved the selection of five interventions for which there was good research evidence of effectiveness and appropriateness but it was known that implementation in clinical practice was poor. At least one intervention was adopted by each of the constituent health authorities in the region.

GRiPP therapeutic interventions[12]

- The use of corticosteroids for women in preterm labour
- The management of services to prevent and treat stroke
- The use of dilatation and curettage for dysfunctional uterine bleeding in women younger than 40 years of age
- The use of grommets in children with chronic otitis media (glue ear)
- Thrombolysis for people with acute myocardial infarction (heart attack).

The main lesson learned from the project was that although much effort was directed at achieving small changes in clinical practice, the impact was far greater on the culture of the organisations. Having a focus on a specific subject for which there was a strong evidence base facilitated the adoption of the change in clinical practice, rather than general exhortations to carry out evidence-based decision making. In addition, the processes of change management and obtaining commitment (as discussed in Chapter 3), the formulation and dissemination of clinical guidelines (Chapters 4 and 5) and evaluation were also essential to the success of the project.

Promoting action on clinical effectiveness (PACE)[13]

This 3-year programme, launched in 1995 by the King's Fund, London, was designed to understand the issues involved in implementing the research findings. The project involved 16 topics within health authorities and trusts, to tackle a range of clinical conditions. The three objectives were to:

- demonstrate effective implementation of evidence-based practice
- develop a national network of individuals interested in clinical effectiveness
- disseminate lessons learnt from local projects.

Some of the key findings concluded:

- that change can be expensive, requiring a significant amount of resources and time
- that existing communication channels should be used as much as possible and that additional meetings should be avoided
- that managing change required a number of different methods – e.g. piloting before 'rolling out', engaging the support of local champions and emphasis on multidisciplinary team development
- careful thought and discussion are required as to which information to collect for monitoring clinical practice early in the life of the project
- local strategies are required for implementing the projects.

Framework for appropriate care throughout Sheffield (FACTS)[14]

This project, which began in 1994, was aimed at general practice and examined the delivery of effective care in three linked clinical areas; aspirin, anti-coagulation and statins. The key lesson from this project was that obtaining an agreement on a topic which was considered worthwhile as a subject for a change in behaviour depended on a number of complex judgements, including:

- whether the issues are perceived as a significant problem by those who have to change
- the extent to which the issue ties in with national policy, and whether it

will be supported by those charged with the task of implementing national policy
- whether all the major problems associated with the change can be solved
- whether there are key individuals or organisations who are strongly opposed to the change
- the nature of the vested interests, either in the proposed change or the *status quo*
- the resource implications of change
- whether there is a significant gap between what people say publicly about the change and what they are actually prepared to do.

One of the main challenges in increasing the uptake of evidence-based practice (and management) in the NHS is the support for this process provided by managers within an organisation. Many of the methods and processes have been discussed in previous chapters.

Support provided by managers to allow the practice of evidence-based care

- Conduct a proper assessment of the main personnel and issues relating to the area to be examined, and work up a robust strategy for achieving change in behaviour
- Allow protected time for clinicians to look up the evidence and have discussions on critical appraisal of the evidence
- Provide funds for specific evidence-based projects
- Ensure that areas to be examined for evidence-based practice are consistent with other obligations of the organisation, including internal and external priorities (e.g. Health Improvement Programmes, other local strategies etc.)
- Ensure that clinicians have access to the evidence (e.g. libraries are open at appropriate times, information from NICE and other relevant organisations is disseminated to clinicians through, for example, a chief knowledge officer)
- Ensure that clinical information systems are appropriate and accessible for use in evidence-based practice
- Ensure access to training on assessing and applying the research
- Encourage clinicians to develop their own personal development plans which reflect their own training needs and are also consistent with the needs of the organisation
- Use the information gleaned from applying the evidence to develop better services
- Ensure that other systems and structures (e.g. clinical audit, clinical risk management and complaints) are interconnected with the process of evidence-based practice.

Purchasers of health care also need to encourage the process through a number of ways, such as:[15]

- The setting up of networks to promote evidence-based practice, share ideas and projects and encourage further research (e.g. the Berkshire Research and Education Network (BREdNet) in Berkshire and the West London Research Network (WeLReN) in West London)
- The identification of resources for clinical governance initiatives and senior professionals nominated to lead initiatives
- The promotion of clinical effectiveness to be the responsibility of all health care managers
- The selection of clinical effectiveness topics to be linked in with service agreement and financial areas
- Monitoring the implementation of evidence-based practice through clinical governance reports.

Issues for consideration

- What management support mechanisms are in place in your organisation to encourage the application of evidence-based practice?
- Do the managers in your organisation get involved actively in such initiatives?

Clinical and health outcomes of care

The end point of good, effective clinical care is that a patient gets better from an acute condition, or that the symptoms of chronic disease are under control. In both cases, the quality of life of the patient should improve so that they are able to carry on with their lives as normally as possible. This end point is known as the outcome of the clinical care or intervention given to a patient for a specific condition.

Of course, the care or intervention a patient receives may be wider than purely clinical in nature; for example, patient self-support no smoking groups, or home help from social services.

Clinical outcomes have been widened into health outcomes. The NHS Executive defines a health outcome as 'the attributable effect of intervention or its lack on a previous health state'.[16]

The assessment of health outcomes is vital, to see if the new intervention or clinical practice has actually improved the health of patients.

Clinical outcomes can be assessed using various aspects of clinical interventions to gauge the effect on patients. Lakhani[17] suggested some clinical interventions which could be used as such measures:

- Avoiding risk of developing disease/ill health
- Reducing risk once it exists
- Early detection and treatment of disease/ill health
- Minimising and managing wider negative consequences of disease/ill health, such as levels of function, disability, handicap, wellbeing, poor quality of life
- Prevention of premature death.

From this, Lakhani identified key questions in assessing the outcomes of interventions:

1. What is the clinical problem?
This question is asked to ensure that clinicians recognise the fact that they have to look further than just the presenting clinical picture of a patient; for example, it is not just the clinical symptoms and signs of angina that matter, it is also the effect of the chest pain on the daily life, work and social activity of patients.

2. What can health services do about the problem?
Clearly, using sound evidence based on research is likely to lead to benefits for patients. The care of patients is provided by a number of health professionals, so a collaborative approach should be used to make decisions about interventions (e.g. through the use of care pathways).

3. What are the objectives of treatment?
This can be illustrated by the range of issues and decisions required when presented with the problem of, for example, the management of chest pain. The objectives of treatment will depend on where the patient is in the possible sequence of events. For example, for someone with mild chest pain on exertion, the objective is to avoid this leading to a myocardial infarction by providing advice on the risk factors for coronary heart disease and prescribing anti-anginal medication. For someone with severe chest pain, the objective is to give the patient thrombolytic therapy to prevent further extension of the cardiac damage.

4. Whose perspective?
There needs to be consideration of the *net* benefit when deciding on a treatment – in other words, the side effects of medication and interventions are weighed up as well as the benefits. Continuing the example of coronary heart disease prevention, a clinician may be concerned about future angina attacks if a patient does not reduce fat intake, whereas the patient may be unable to change his or her diet because somebody else cooks the food, or because there are cultural differences in diet (for example, it is no good giving an Asian diabetic a western diet sheet to follow).

5. What services are required?

It is relatively simple to specify the services and interventions once the objectives are clear. However, if a whole range of interventions is required over a period of time, this may involve a number of professionals in the health service and even outside it. For example, cardiac rehabilitation after myocardial infarction can be initiated while in hospital and good progress made as a result, but this may not continue if there are no services in the community to support this treatment.

6. What are the standards?

The chances of achieving better outcomes are improved if the services delivering them do so to specified standards. Guidelines are an obvious vehicle for this (see Chapters 4 and 5).

7. What are the results?

Here, the question is whether the desired results have been achieved, and whether this was because of clinical action. Clinical audit can help answer this (see Chapter 5).

An alternative view comes from the Health Outcomes Institute in the USA, which suggested that patient outcomes can be put into seven categories:

1. Clinical – the medical measures of blood pressure, size and shape of tumours, blood levels of various chemicals and drugs and so on
2. Death – the mortality from all types of causes
3. Disease – long-term conditions and diseases likely to affect normal functioning
4. Functional status – measures of what people are able to do (e.g. walk unaided, climb up stairs etc.)
5. Wellbeing – the emotional and mental state of patients, including the degree of pain
6. Satisfaction – the perception by patients of their own care
7. Cost – both direct and indirect.

Sometimes it is not possible to assess the outcome of an intervention directly because the end point is difficult to measure or the time scales are too long for the particular situation that is being considered. Another approach is to look at system outcomes. These are measures to see if a new system is working well and meeting its own set of targets; for example, a target could be to have 90% of people with suspected myocardial infarction admitted to the coronary care unit within an hour of attendance at A&E. If that is achieved, then it is possible to conclude that the system is effective. This type of measure is sometimes called a performance or key indicator.

Clinical indicators are incorporated into the NHS Performance Indicators, which are measures used to help NHS organisations monitor the delivery of health services against plans for improvement.[18] These have been discussed further in Chapter 1.

The demonstration of evidence-based management is still in its infancy; however, there have been examples of its effective application as discussed above. The challenges in the future for managers, as for clinicians, are to apply this evidence more systematically, to learn from previous initiatives (and mistakes) and to work with clinical colleagues to achieve this aim.

References

1. Muir Gray J A 1997 Evidence-based healthcare: how to make health policy decisions and management decisions. Churchill Livingstone, Edinburgh
2. Mintzberg H 1973 The nature of managerial work. Harper and Row, London
3. Mullins L J 1996 Management and organisational behaviour, 4th edn. Pitman Publishing, London
4. Stewart R 1983 Choices for the manager. McGraw-Hill, London
5. The Institute of Health Services Management 1998 Statement of primary values. IHSM, London
6. Wright J, Williams R, Wilkinson J R 1998 Development and the importance of health needs assessment. British Medical Journal 316: 1310-1313
7. Simnet I 1995 Managing health promotion: developing health organisations and communities. John Wiley and Son, Chichester
8. Health Education Authority 1995 Promoting physical activity: guidance for commissioners, purchasers and providers. Health Education Authority, London
9. Johnstone P, Zolese G 1999 Systematic review of the effectiveness of planned short hospital stays for mental healthcare. British Medical Journal 318: 1387-1390
10. Griffin S 1998 Diabetes care in general practice: meta-analysis of randomised controlled trials. British Medical Journal 317: 390-396
11. Whitfield L 1999 Taking the stand [news focus]. Health Service Journal 17th June: 13-15
12. Dunning M, McQuay H, Milne R 1994 Getting a GRiP. Health Service Journal 5400 28th April; 104: 24-26
13. Dunning M, Abi-Aad G, Gilbert D et al 1999 Experience, evidence and everyday practice. King's Fund Publishing, London
14. Eve R, Golton I, Hodgkin P et al 1997 Learning from the framework for appropriate care throughout Sheffield (FACTS) project. University of Sheffield, Sheffield
15. Johnston P, Wright J [in press] Promoting evidence-based practice through commissioning: results of a national workshop
16. NHS Executive 1996 Promoting clinical effectiveness: a framework for action in and through the NHS. NHS Executive, London
17. Lakhani A 1995 The role of outcomes assessment in improving clinical effectiveness. In: Deighan M, Hitch S (eds) Clinical Effectiveness: Guidelines to

cost-effective practice. Earlybrave Publications Limited, Brentwood
18. NHS Executive 2000 Improving quality and performance in the new NHS: NHS performance indicators. Health Service Circular 2000/023

10

Some legal and ethical principles

The process of clinical governance cannot operate sensibly without reference to some legal and ethical principles. This chapter discusses some of these principles and raises some issues pertinent to clinical governance.

Ethical principles

It was Hippocrates in 400 BC who first developed a concept which is now reflected in the principles of clinical governance and based upon self-regulation.

It is a popular misconception that all newly qualified doctors go through the ritual of swearing upon the Hippocratic Oath when they emerge from medical school having been through 5 or so years of training. In reality, medical ethics is taught in a patchy manner in medical schools up and down the country, and much of what determines and influences the conduct of a doctor is picked up after qualification. However, the principles of medical ethics are based on areas of conduct that few would argue with:

- to preserve life
- to alleviate suffering
- to do no harm
- to tell the truth
- to respect the patient's autonomy
- to deal justly with patients.

There may be occasions, however, when these principles conflict. For example, surgery to alleviate a bowel obstruction is not without risk from the anaesthetic, but the benefits may outweigh this risk. The analysis of the balance between risk and benefits is required for most health care interventions, to varying degrees. Furthermore, in a situation of limited resources and major advances in health care technology and drugs, ethical clinicians must also pay attention to costs, as the decision to devote resources to one patient has the effect of denying them to another. This balance between cost and benefits must also be considered by clinical decision-makers.

Looking at health care delivery on a more global level, managers and clinicians are faced with a number of ethical issues including:

- the increasing rate of consumption of resources due to increasing demand
- the limited resources available for health care require decisions about who is to have access to care and the type and extent of coverage
- the complexity and cost of the health care delivery system may cause a tension between what is good for society as a whole and what is best for an individual patient
- flaws in health care delivery systems may cause those working in the system to manipulate it for the benefit of a specific patient or segment of a population rather than to work for the improvement of the delivery of care to all. This exacerbates the flaws and produces a downward spiral.

Various professional and regulatory bodies have issued codes of conduct to guide their members; however, it seems that only the code of conduct produced jointly between the NHS Confederation and the Institute of Healthcare Management for NHS managers makes a reference to the use of resources in the best interests of the public and patients.[1] And so the seeds of potential and actual conflict are sown concerning access to health care and decisions around the rationing of care.

Duties of a doctor registered with the General Medical Council[2]

Patients must be able to trust doctors with their lives and wellbeing. To justify that trust, we as a profession have a duty to maintain a good standard of practice and care and to show respect for human life. In particular as a doctor you must:

- make the care of your patient your first concern
- treat every patient politely and considerately
- respect patients' dignity and privacy
- listen to patients and respect their views
- give patients information in a way they can understand
- respect the rights of patients to be fully involved in decisions about their care
- keep your professional knowledge and skills up-to-date
- recognise the limits of your professional competence

- be honest and trustworthy
- respect and protect confidential information
- make sure that your personal beliefs do not prejudice your patients' care
- act quickly to protect patients from risk if you have good reason to believe that you or a colleague may not be fit to practise
- avoid abusing your position as a doctor
- work with colleagues in the ways that best serve patients' interests.

In all these matters you must never discriminate unfairly against your patients or colleagues. And you must always be prepared to justify your actions to them.

Code of conduct for NHS managers[1]

The code encapsulates the key duties expected of NHS managers and should form the basis of every manager's day-to-day duties.

As an NHS manager, I will observe the following principles:

- make the care and safety of patients my first concern and act to protect them from risk
- respect the public, patients, relatives, carers, NHS staff and partners in other agencies
- be honest and act with integrity
- accept responsibility for my own work and the proper performance of the people I manage
- show my commitment to working as a team member by working with all my colleagues in the NHS and the wider community
- take responsibility for my own learning and development.

This means in particular that:

1. I will:
- respect patient confidentiality
- use the resources available to me in an effective, efficient and timely manner having proper regard to the best interests of the public and patients
- be guided by the interests of the patients while ensuring a safe working environment
- act to protect patients from risk by putting into practice appropriate support and disciplinary procedures for staff
- seek to ensure that anyone with a genuine concern is treated reasonably and fairly.

2. I will respect and treat with dignity and fairness, the public, patients, relatives, carers, NHS staff and partners in other agencies. In my capacity as a senior manager within the NHS I will seek to ensure that no one is unlawfully discriminated against

because of their religion, belief, race, colour, gender, marital status, sexual orientation, disability, age, social and economic status or national origin. I will also seek to ensure that:

- the public are properly informed and able to influence service provision
- patients are informed about and involved in their own care, their experience is valued and they are involved in decisions
- relatives and carers are, with the consent of patients, involved in the care of their relatives and the people they care for
- NHS staff are valued as colleagues, properly informed about the management of the NHS, given appropriate opportunities to participate in decision making, given all reasonable protection from harassment and bullying, provided with a safe working environment, helped to maintain and improve their knowledge and skills and fulfil their potential. NHS staff should be enabled to achieve a reasonable work/personal life balance
- Partners in other agencies are invited to make their contribution to improving health and health services.

3. I will be honest and act with integrity and probity at all times. I will not make, permit or knowingly allow to be made, any untrue or misleading statement relating to my own duties or the functions of my employer. I will seek to ensure that:

- the best interests of the public and patients/clients are upheld in decision making and that decisions are not influenced by gifts and inducements
- NHS resources are protected from fraud and corruption and that any incident of this kind is reported to the NHS Counter Fraud Services
- judgements about colleagues (including appraisals and references) are consistent, fair and unbiased and are properly founded
- open and learning organisations are created in which concerns about people breaking the Code can be raised without fear.

4. I will accept responsibility for my own work and the proper performance of the people I manage. I will seek to ensure that those I manage accept that they are responsible for their own actions to:

- the public and their representatives by explaining and justifying the use of resources and the performance of the NHS
- patients, relatives and carers by answering questions and complaints in an open, honest and well researched way and in a manner which provides a full explanation of what has happened and of what will be done to deal with poor performance and, where appropriate, giving an apology
- NHS staff and partners in other agencies by explaining and justifying decisions on the use of resources and give due and proper consideration to suggestions for improving performance, the use of resources and service delivery.

I will support and assist the Accountable Officer of my organisation in his/her responsibility to answer to Parliament, Ministers and the Department of Health in terms of fully and faithfully declaring and explaining the use of resources and the performance of the local NHS in putting national policy into practice and delivering targets.

For the avoidance of doubt, nothing in paragraphs 2-4 of this Code requires or authorises an NHS manager to whom this Code applies to:

- make, commit or knowingly allow to be made any unlawful disclosure
- make, permit or knowingly allow to be made any disclosure in breach of his/her duties and obligations to his/her employer save as permitted by law.

If there is any conflict between the above duties and obligations and this Code, the former shall prevail.

5. I will show my commitment to team working by creating an environment in which:
- teams of front line staff are able to work together in the best interests of patients
- leadership is encouraged and developed at all levels and in all staff groups
- the NHS plays its full part in community development.

6. I will take responsibility for my own learning and development. I will seek to:
- take full advantage of the opportunities provided
- keep up-to-date with best practice
- share my learning and development with others.

Nursing and Midwifery Council Code of Professional Conduct[3]

As a registered nurse or midwife, you are personally accountable for your practice. In caring for patients and clients you must:
- respect the patient or client as an individual
- obtain consent before you give any treatment or care
- protect confidential information
- co-operate with others in the team
- maintain your professional knowledge and competence
- be trustworthy
- act to identify and minimise risk to patients and clients.

The professional codes of conducts for clinicians are binding and if these are breached in any way, then the right to practise may be withheld from the practitioner concerned. For NHS managers, if they break their code of conduct, they will lose their jobs and will not be allowed to work in the NHS again.

In an attempt to develop a shared statement of ethical principles, a group convened by the *British Medical Journal*, called the Tavistock Group, set upon a task to try to bring together all stakeholders in health care into a more consistent moral framework, to engender co-operative behaviour and mutual respect. The aim was to develop a unified code of ethics relevant to all professionals involved in the delivery of health care and to map out strategies for implementing the code.

The first joint statement of health care principles was produced in 1999. Its aim was to heighten awareness of the need for principles to guide all those involved in the delivery of health care. The focus is on the direction of health care delivery systems, which should be on the service of individuals and the good of society as a whole, whilst providing a basis for enhanced co-operation amongst all involved (e.g. health care professionals, health care agencies, other organisations including insurers, employers and government and the public).

The statement declares that five major principles should govern health care systems:[4]

1. Health care is a human right.
2. The care of individuals is at the centre of health care delivery, but must be viewed and practised within the overall context of continuing work to generate the greatest possible health gains for groups and populations.
3. The responsibilities of the health care delivery system must include the prevention of illness and the alleviation of disability.
4. Co-operation with each other and those served is imperative for those working within the health care delivery system.
5. All individuals and groups involved in health care, whether providing access or services, have the continuing responsibility to help improve its quality.

It is worth noting that, although the last principle makes a reference to the continuous improvement of the quality of care (thereby echoing the requirements of clinical governance), the issue of managing within existing resources seems to have been side stepped. The latter is covered by the implementation of the Human Rights Act 1998 which states that a public body may, in certain circumstances, no longer be able to use the excuse of a lack of money to withhold or limit a particular treatment.

Issues for consideration

Consider the following scenarios:

- A community mental health team has been caring for a woman who suffers from chronic schizophrenia for 3 years. The black and Asian members of the team have been constantly at the receiving end of racist comments from the woman's relatives. The team is torn. They do not wish to have contact with the patient, but they know they provide care 'above and beyond' in an effort to combat any adverse comment. They are also aware that the woman is vulnerable.

- A primary care group is asked to consider the funding of new drug treatment for rheumatoid arthritis which will stop the progression of the disease at an early stage for a young patient. This patient fits the profile of the type of patient for whom the drug proved beneficial in trials. The PCG is already running a deficit and this is before the heavy winter season starts.

How can the joint statement of health care principles help in these situations?

Ethical matters do not usually have easy or straightforward answers when applied to day-to-day situations; however, there are some legal principles that do provide a guide as to how clinical care should be provided. This is based on an assessment of competence in health care.

Legal principles

The following is not intended as a comprehensive analysis of the law. Rather, it is a discussion of some of the basic principles, using extracts from cases and guidelines where appropriate. The discussion is confined to the relationship between the health care professional and the patient, and does not cover the ethical/human rights issues involved in rationing access to health care.

The Human Rights Act 1998

In October 2000, the Human Rights Act 1998 came into force, bringing the European Convention on Human Rights into UK law.[5] The Convention was drafted by British lawyers and adopted as a collective response to the horrors of the Second World War by the countries of Europe.[6] The rights are not all absolute (except for Article 3), and apply to both individuals and companies. Some rights are qualified by specific exceptions, such as the rights to life and liberty (Articles 2 and 5 respectively) – for example, people can be detained lawfully if they are of unsound mind. Other rights require broader interpretation – for example, the right to respect for private life (Article 8). Here, there will be instances of the state being allowed to restrict this right and judges will need to balance the interests of the individual against those of the wider community.

The rights of humans[6]

- Article 2 – The right to life
- Article 3 – The prohibition of torture and inhuman degrading treatment
- Article 4 – The prohibition of slavery
- Article 5 – The right to liberty
- Article 6 – The right to a fair trial
- Article 7 – No retrospective crimes
- Article 8 – The right to respect for private and family life, home and correspondence
- Article 9 – The freedom of thought, conscience and religion
- Article 10 – The freedom of expression and right to information
- Article 11 – The freedom of assembly and association
- Article 12 – The right to marry and found a family
- Article 14 – The freedom from discrimination in respect of protected rights

NB – Article 1 was not included in the Act and there are additional rights relating to the right to property, the right to education and the right to free elections.

All public bodies, including the NHS and local authorities, have a statutory duty to act compatibly with human rights. If people consider that their rights have been violated, they are now able to bring proceedings and claim damages. Judges are obliged to interpret laws in the context of the Human Rights Act when considering disputes between the state and individuals.

Further information on the Human Rights Act and how it relates to the UK health service can be obtained from www.doh.gov.uk/humanrights.

Legal competence in health care

In practice the issue of competence in health care tends to focus on the issue of negligence, and in many legal cases the central point is one of causation. To establish legal liability, a claimant needs to demonstrate that a legal duty of care was owed by the health care practitioner to the patient; that there was a breach of that duty; and that injury was caused by the breach. Both a breach of duty (or negligence) and causation must be present for there to be liability.

Duty

The duty of care can arise between a health care practitioner and patient, and applies to anyone who is, or purports to be, skilled in medical matters and who treats a patient, so it includes, for example, paramedics and practitioners in complementary medicine, etc. It applies to all clinical treatment.

Breach of duty

The duty of care is breached if the practitioner provides care that falls below a standard of practice accepted by a responsible body of medical opinion. This is known as the Bolam test.[7] In this situation, the court takes advice from medical or nursing experts in the relevant clinical speciality in order to determine what the ordinary skilled doctor or nurse in that speciality would have been expected to do when faced with the circumstances of the case. Like is compared with like – for example, a junior doctor in radiology facing an allegation of missing a fracture will be judged by the standard of a junior doctor in radiology, and not by the standard of a consultant in radiology. The state of medical science is taken as that relating to the date of the alleged negligence and not the date of the court hearing.

The judge in the *Bolam v. Friern Hospital Management Committee* (1957) case said:

> The test is the standard of the ordinary skilled man exercising and professing to have that special skill. A man need not possess the highest expert skill; it is well-established law that it is sufficient if he exercises the ordinary skill of an ordinary competent man exercising that particular art.

> A doctor is not guilty of negligence if he has acted in accordance with a practice accepted as proper by a responsible body of medical men skilled in that particular article. Putting it the other way round, a doctor is not negligent if he is acting in accordance with such a practice, merely because there is a body of opinion that takes a contrary view. At the same time, that does not mean that a medical man can obstinately and pig-headedly carry on with some old technique if it has been proved to be contrary to what is really substantially the whole of informed medical opinion.

The phrase 'responsible body of medical opinion' has been emphasised more recently. In *Bolitho v. City and Hackney HA* (1997),[8] the House of Lords said that in very rare cases, the court could reject the opinion of a body of medical opinion if it was not reasonable, or responsible.

> The court is not bound to hold that a defendant doctor escapes liability for negligent treatment or diagnosis just because he leads evidence from a number of experts who are genuinely of the opinion that the defendant's treatment or diagnosis accorded with sound medical practice... The use of these adjectives – responsible, reasonable and respectable [in Bolam and Maynard] – all show that the court has to be satisfied that the exponents of the body of opinion relied upon can demonstrate that such opinion has a logical basis. In particular, in cases involving, as they often do, the weighing of risks against benefits, the judge before accepting a body of opinion as being responsible, reasonable or respectable, will need to be satisfied that, in forming their views, the experts have directed their minds to the question of comparative risks and benefits and have reached a defensible conclusion on the matter.

Expert evidence of what is good practice, as accepted by a responsible body, may be substantiated by the use of evidence-based clinical guidelines that have been carefully put together in the manner discussed in Chapter 5. However, the judgement also says that doctors and nurses have a legally recognised discretion to follow their own clinical judgement provided it is reasonable. Blind adherence without questioning the appropriateness of the guidelines in particular situations may be evidence of negligence if the treatment is inappropriate for the individual patient.

The Bolam/Bolitho principle forms the basis on which the standard of clinical care is judged by the courts.

Provided there is a substantial body of reasonable of medical opinion in favour of a particular practice, then negligence will not be established.

Causation

The claimant must show that the negligence caused injury and loss. This is frequently the most difficult area in a medical negligence case because, in some cases, the patient's health would have deteriorated even if the treatment were competent. The nature of the claimant's clinical condition and past medical history also needs to be taken into account.

Three night watchmen presented to A&E with continuous vomiting after drinking tea. The triage nurse relayed the complaint to the casualty doctor, who told them to go home and call their own GPs. One of them died a few hours later. The Court of Appeal held the casualty doctor negligent, but there was no liability, due to lack of causation. It was found that death was due to arsenic poisoning, for which there was no reasonable prospect of providing an antidote.[9] In other words, the night watchman would probably have died even if treatment had been administered in hospital – it was not the negligence that caused the death.

Competence and consent to treatment

The NHS Plan recognised the need for a more robust approach to obtaining consent from patients[10] so that their needs are taken properly into account when deciding on treatment options. A reference guide to consent for examination or treatment was published in 2001[11] in order to provide guidance on English law concerning consent to physical interventions on patients. The guidance is relevant to all health professionals, including students, and takes into account the Human Rights Act 1998.

The Reference Guide to Consent for Examination or Treatment covers the following areas:[12]

- The process of seeking consent, who should seek consent and what to do when consent is withdrawn or refused.
- The procedure to be followed in adults without capacity, e.g. those under sedation or anaesthetic or those who have a long-standing incapacity and, where there is doubt, when to refer to the courts for a decision on capacity.
- The process to follow with children and young people under the age of 18, and the concept of 'Gillick competence' when a child has sufficient understanding and intelligence to consent to an intervention without necessarily needing the consent of a person with parental responsibility.
- The principles applicable to withdrawing and withholding life-prolonging treatment to adults and children with capacity, and those lacking capacity, and in situations of brain stem death.

The guidance sets the exceptions to the principles detailed above:
- Part IV of the Mental Health Act sets out the circumstances in which patients detained under the Act may be treated without consent for their mental disorder; however, it does not apply to treatment for physical conditions unrelated to the psychiatric problem. The reforms proposed in the White Paper Reforming the Mental Health Act published in December 2000 do not affect this principle.13
- The Public Health (Control of Disease) Act 1984 states that people who have certain notifiable infectious diseases can be medically examined, removed to, and detained in a hospital without their consent.
- Section 47 of the National Assistance Act 1948 states that people who have a grave chronic disease, are old, infirm or physically disabled and are living in insanitary conditions can be removed to more suitable premises for care and attention.

There is other guidance which details the processes to be followed when seeking consent from children,[14] older people[15] and people with learning disabilities.[16] There are also gudes for patients on what they have a right to expect on consent.[17]

Model policy and consent documents which contain a core minimum of information have been issued in order to ensure consistency of approach to obtaining consent from patients across the NHS in England.[18] In addition, good practice states that the person who is seeking the consent ideally should be the one who is treating the patient. It is possible, however, to obtain consent on behalf of a colleague if the person seeking the consent is capable of performing the procedure in question or has been specially trained to seek consent for that procedure.

Individual NHS trusts are required to produce a consent to treatment policy based on the model document, and should state the conditions under which written, as opposed to oral, consent to treatment is necessary and what form of consent is appropriate for specific procedures.

The requirements of the consent procedures mean that clinicians need more rigorous training in communication skills to ensure that key points are discussed with patients concerning the treatment they are receiving, so that the consent given is as well-informed as possible. Interpreters who have specific training to seek consent appropriately are also required for patients who do not speak English.

Model consent forms[19]

1. Consent form 1: for patients able to consent for themselves
2. Consent form 2: for those with parental responsibility, consenting on behalf of a child or young person
3. Consent form 3: both for patients able to consent for themselves and for those with parental responsibility consenting on behalf of a child/young person, where the procedure does not involve any impairment of consciousness. The use of the form is optional
4. Consent form 4: for use where the patient is an adult unable to consent to investigation or treatment
5. Consent form on the taking and use of human organs and tissue from post mortem examinations.[20]

The consent form should explain:

- the nature and effect of treatment
- major and characteristic risks
- any other procedures which may become necessary during treatment, and available alternatives
- type of anaesthetic used.

Seeking consent

It is an important principle to note, that in relation to any type of treatment or examination, from major surgery, to blood tests to anaesthesia, English law clearly states that one adult cannot give consent to an intervention on behalf of another adult. Consent can be given, however, for the treatment of children.

In order for consent to be valid, it must be given voluntarily by a person who is appropriately informed (the patient or, where relevant, someone with a parental responsibility for a patient under the age of 18). This person must have the capacity to consent to the intervention concerned.

Assessing capacity

The capacity of a patient to understand is assessed using the following criteria:[21]

- the ability to comprehend and retain information about treatment
- the ability to believe information
- the ability to weigh the information and make a decision.

The test case was that of a schizophrenic man who refused an amputation for a gangrenous leg which could have threatened his life. He was judged to be competent because he understood and believed the risks of refusing the treatment, and was able to make a balanced decision to consent to it, or not. The treatment was not provided, and he survived.[21]

> A competent patient is of sound mind, capable of understanding the nature of the proposed treatment.
>
> An incompetent patient is incapable of understanding, or unconscious, but does not necessarily fall within the definition of the Mental Health Act 1983.[22]

In the case of adults who are not competent to give consent, the law permits treatment of that person if it would be in their best interests. Note, however, that this is not the same as consent being given by someone else. The concept of 'best interests' includes a wide variety of factors such as the wishes and beliefs of the patient when competent, their current wishes and their general wellbeing, including spiritual and religious welfare.

At any point in their treatment, patients can withdraw their consent, even during the performance of a procedure. If that situation occurs, it is good practice for the health professional to stop the procedure, if possible, establish the patient's concerns and explain the consequences of not continuing with the treatment.

Clear written notes in the patient's records provide an important account of the discussions concerning consent.

Consent: adults

The general principle with adults is that every competent patient has a right to decide what should be done with his/her body. It is appropriate for an adult to refuse treatment if:[23]

- the patient's capacity has not been diminished by illness, medication, false assumptions or misinformation
- the patient is not being unduly influenced by a third party
- the circumstances in which the patient made the decision have not changed.

If there are any doubts concerning the validity of a refusal for essential treatment in a life-threatening situation, an application should be made to the court for a declaration.

Consent: children

For children under 16 years of age, parental consent is required for examination or treatment, unless the child is capable of providing valid consent. The final decision, however, is based on the principle that the welfare of the child is paramount. The parent has no automatic veto on treatment which is in a child's best interests. Nor can they consent to treatment which is not in the child's best interests. Where there is a dispute, a court order may have to be sought and the court will hear evidence from the parents and the clinicians on the medical issues of each case.

To be eligible to give consent, a parent must have parental responsibility under the Children Act 1989. In the case of married parents, both have the responsibility if married at the time of birth; for unmarried parents, the mother alone has the responsibility. For married parents, one or the other or both can give consent, whereas for unmarried parents, the father has to obtain a parental responsibility by court order or a parental responsibility agreement under the Act. If there is a conflict between married parents, or if they refuse consent, a specific issues order should be obtained under Section 8 of the Children's Act 1989.

There needs to be careful consideration of the validity of a child's consent or refusal. If a doctor is satisfied that a child under the age of 16 has sufficient understanding of a proposed examination or treatment to give a valid consent, then this can proceed. This is known as Gillick competence[24] after a case of the same name. A parent cannot override a Gillick-competent child's consent, but it can be overridden by the court.

For Gillick competent children:

- a full record should be made in the child's notes of the factors taken into account when assessing the child's understanding of a proposed examination or treatment
- efforts should be made, if a child is seen alone, to persuade them to inform their parents, unless it is clearly not in their interest to do so.

Jehovah's witnesses

Jehovah's witnesses refuse the use of blood or blood products for medical treatment. Competent adults can refuse consent to treatment, even though its refusal may cause their death. It is important to assess competence very carefully, and if there is any doubt, an application should be made to the court. For children, a court order should be sought. The court will usually make an order for treatment if it is in the best interests of the child, and if the situation is life threatening.

Persistent vegetative state

This issue was first brought to prominence in a case involving a young man called Tony Bland who was crushed at the Hillsborough football stadium disaster and had been in a persistent vegetative state for 4 years. It was declared by the House of Lords that treatment could lawfully be withheld, even though it would lead to his death, because the continuation of treatment was not in his best interests. Both the hospital and his parents supported the application.

The outcome of the Tony Bland case was that:[25]

- euthanasia by a positive step to end life is unlawful
- doctors should apply to the court for a declaration before withholding medical treatment in a cases of a persistent vegetative state
- medical treatment could lawfully be withheld where further treatment is not in the patient's best interests, there is no hope of recovery and the patient will shortly die, provided that responsible medical opinion feels that continuing treatment is futile.

The same legal principles apply to withdrawing and withholding life-prolonging treatment as apply to any other medical intervention, which includes the use of artificial nutrition and hydration.

It is important to distinguish between withdrawing or withholding treatment which is of no clinical benefit to the patient or is not in the patient's best interests, and taking deliberate action to end the person's life.

The British Medical Association has issued some guidance on withholding and withdrawing life-prolonging medical treatment[26] in response to the increasing ability of medical technology to sustain life. The guidelines propose a number of steps to making the decision:

1. The doctor must first judge against a set of criteria whether a patient is benefiting from being kept alive

2. If there is no benefit, then a second opinion should be sought from a senior clinician with experience in the condition from which the patient is suffering but who has no personal connection with the case
3. The doctor should then involve the whole health care team in discussion and the decision
4. The family must also be involved in the final decision; in particular, the doctor should seek guidance on what the patient would have most wanted
5. If the family cannot be persuaded that it is time to withdraw treatment, then an application can be made to the courts
6. The guidelines also say that parents must be involved in cases of babies and very young children who have no chance of a viable life. Dying or very ill patients who ask not to be treated and those who have left an advanced directive refusing life-prolonging treatment should have their wishes respected.

Factors that determine whether a treatment will benefit a patient[26]

- The patient's own wishes and values (where these can be ascertained)
- Clinical judgement about the effectiveness of the proposed treatment and the likelihood of the patient experiencing severe, unmanageable pain or suffering
- The level of awareness the individual has of his or her existence or surroundings, as demonstrated by an ability to interact somehow with others and/or an ability to take control of any aspect of his or her life
- The likelihood and extent of any improvement in the patient's condition if the treatment is provided, and whether the invasiveness of the treatment is justified in the circumstances
- The views of the parents if the patient is a child
- The views of people close to the patient, especially close relations, partners and carers, about what the patient is likely to see as beneficial.

Ms B, a 43-year-old professional woman, had a haemorrhage in a cavernous haemangioma in her upper spinal cord. Following an almost complete recovery she had another haemorrhage 2 years later which left her quadriplegic and dependent on artificial ventilation. She was advised to consider specialist rehabilitation after review by experts who said that she had negligible chance of substantial recovery. Ms B, after investigating extensively her prognosis, requested to have her ventilation discontinued as she felt that her quality of life was intolerable as she was very dependent on others and she had little control over her own body. The clinicians felt unable to carry out her request and Ms B took the NHS trust treating her to court. The judge ruled in her favour, saying that:

A mentally competent patient has an absolute right to refuse to consent to treatment for any reason, rational or irrational, or for no reason at all, even where that decision may lead to his or her own death.

Furthermore, the judgment also highlighted that:
The right of the competent patient to request cessation of treatment must prevail over the natural desire of the medical and nursing professions to try to keep her alive.[27]

Although the doctor can 'withdraw' treatment that is either refused or no longer in the patient's best interests, he or she may never take active steps to hasten a patient's death. To do so could amount to murder.

Living wills

There is an increasing movement by some people to make their wishes known in advance concerning future medical treatment (including the withdrawal of feeding and/or hydration) in the event of their becoming incompetent. This is known as a living will (and also known as advance directive, advance decision, advance statement, advance consent or advance refusal). Provided that the patient was of capacity when the living will was made, and understood the circumstances in which it may operate, then the living will has to be followed. An advance refusal is valid if made voluntarily by a person, appropriately informed, with capacity.

Incompetent patients

This situation may be applicable to people who are not being considered for treatment under the Mental Health Act 1983, and in the treatment of mentally disordered patients for conditions other than their mental illness.

Mental disorder is defined as mental illness, arrested or incomplete development of the mind, psychopathic disorder, and any other disorder or disability of the mind.[28]

In normal circumstances the clinician will apply the 'best interests' test as defined by the case *re: F.*[29] Care is needed when considering treatment for incompetent patients and the following precautions should be taken:[22]

- A detailed record should be made in the patient's records as to why the patient is considered to be incapable and why the proposed treatment is in his/her best interests. This should be discussed with another, preferably more senior, doctor who should countersign the records.
- It is considered good practice to consult with the relatives, although this does raise issues of confidentiality.

- The patient's capabilities must be judged at the time of treatment, as incompetence can be transitory.
- In a situation where a patient is under anaesthetic and the surgeon discovers the need to perform a procedure for which consent has not been obtained, the surgeon should proceed with caution and do the minimum necessary to deal with the circumstances. However, it may be necessary to delay the procedure until the appropriate consent has been obtained. Ideally, the surgeon should carry out a full discussion with the patient if it is anticipated that there may be a need for a further procedure.

Resuscitation

The primary goal of medical treatment is to benefit patients, and prolonging a patient's life usually provides that benefit. However, it is not appropriate for medical care to prolong life at any cost with no regard to its quality, or to the burdens of treatment on the patient. Mentally competent may reach a stage at which they feel that further treatment to prolong their life would no longer be acceptable. The NHS Executive has produced guidance on discussing and developing resuscitation policies so that patients' rights are respected in this matter.[30] The guidance has been based on the joint statement from the British Medical Association, the Resuscitation Council (UK) and the Royal College of Nursing, Decisions Relating to Cardiopulmonary Resuscitation (CPR).[31]

The statement highlights a number of issues, including:[31]

Principles

- Timely support for patients and people close to them, and effective, sensitive communication are essential
- Decisions must be based on the individual patient's circumstances and reviewed regularly
- Sensitive advance discussion should always be encouraged, but not forced
- Information about CPR and the chances of a successful outcome need to be realistic.

Practical matters

- Information about CPR policies should be displayed for patients and staff
- Leaflets should be available for patients and people close to them explaining about CPR, how decisions are made and their involvement in decisions

- Decisions about attempting CPR must be communicated effectively to relevant health professionals.

In emergencies

- If no advance decision has been made or is known, CPR should be attempted unless:
  - The patient has refused CPR
  - The patient is clearly in the terminal phase of illness; or
  - The burdens of treatment outweigh the benefits.

Advance decision making

- Competent patients should be involved in discussions about attempting CPR unless they indicate that they do not want to be
- Where patients lack competence to participate, people close to them can be helpful in reflecting their views.

Legal issues

- Patients' rights under the Human Rights Act must be taken into account in decision making
- Neither patients nor relatives can demand treatment which the health care team judges to be inappropriate, but all efforts will be made to accommodate wishes and preferences
- In England, Wales and Northern Ireland relatives and people close to the patient are not entitled in law to take health care decisions for the patient
- In Scotland, adults may appoint a health care proxy to give consent to medical treatment
- Health professionals need to be aware of the law in relation to decision making for children and young people.

For a mentally impaired person, the court should be asked to consider whether a do not resuscitate policy is appropriate.

Pregnant women

Can a pregnant woman give a competent consent or refusal? This is a difficult area, but the position is that the wishes of the competent mother cannot be overruled in favour of the rights of the unborn child, because the child has no legal rights which contradict the mother's right to refuse treatment. The situation currently is that it is pointless to apply for a declaration to the High Court if the patient is competent. Trusts should, for their own protection, seek unequivocal assurances from the patient, recorded in writing, that a refusal was a result of an informed decision.

Public interest disclosure

Both the GMC and the NMC codes of professional conduct make reference to drawing attention to the appropriate authorities if the practice of a colleague is felt to be detrimental to patients. This, however, has sometimes resulted in the 'whistle blower' being suspended, disciplined and/or losing his or her job and status.

On 2 July 1999, a new law was introduced to protect employees in the United Kingdom who 'blow the whistle' on wrong doing or malpractice at work, called the Public Interest Disclosure Act 1998. This private member's bill enables employees, including NHS staff (doctors, nurses and professionals allied to medicine) and contract and agency staff to raise concerns about poor or dangerous practice without endangering their own careers.

All NHS organisations are required to draw up and implement whistle blowing policies. NHS staff are required, in the first instance, to raise concerns through their employers or the Department of Health. If robust evidence can substantiate the concern, disclosure to regulators, including the National Audit Office and the Health and Safety Executive, will be protected. In some limited circumstances, even disclosure to the media will be safeguarded.

The law aims to protect whistle blowers from sacking or victimisation. Employment tribunals have the power to 'freeze' a dismissal and make unlimited compensation awards.

Issues for consideration

Dr Stephen Bolsin, consultant anaesthetist, spent 5 years trying to draw attention to the unsatisfactory standards of paediatric cardiac surgery at Bristol Royal Infirmary Trust during the early 1990s. He now works in Australia. Professor Peter Dawson had to resign after raising concerns about the out-of-hours cover in the radiology department at the Hammersmith Hospitals Trust.

Both have expressed caution concerning how the change in behaviour can be brought about by the change in the law on whistle blowing.

- How does this legal protection operate in your organisation?

Conclusions

Clinical governance has an important role to play in improving the public's confidence in the delivery and quality of health care. The trust that patients and carers place in health professionals needs to be supported by knowledge that the treatment is evidence-based and effective, and that the clinical staff are appropriately trained. Many of the processes supporting the clinical governance framework were in place prior to the statutory duty being formally established. The challenge is to draw current good practice under one umbrella, and to develop the new systems alongside in such a way as to make it open and accessible to the public whilst being supportive to health care staff.

References
1. NHS Executive 2002 Code of conduct for NHS managers. The Stationery Office, London
2. General Medical Council 1995 Good medical practice: guidance from the General Medical Council. GMC Publications, London
3. Nursing and Midwifery Council 2002 Code of professional conduct. NMC, London
4. Scott H 1999 Code crackers. Health Management June: 19-21
5. Human rights act 1998. The Stationery Office, London
6. Hewson B 2000 Why the human rights act matters to doctors. British Medical Journal 321: 780-781
7. Bolam v Friern Hospital Management Committee [1957] 2 All ER 635
8. Bolitho v City and Hackney HA [1997] 4 All ER 771
9. Barnett v Chelsea and Kensington Hospital Management Committee [1968] 1 All ER 1068
10. Department of Health 2000 The NHS plan: a plan for investment, a plan for reform. The Stationery Office, London
11. Department of Health 2001 Reference guide to consent for examination or treatment. The Stationery Office, London
12. Swage T 2002 The new consent procedures. Health Service Manager Briefing 79, 13 May
13. Department of Health and Home Office 2000 Reforming the mental health act. The Stationery Office, London
14. Department of Health 2001 Seeking consent: working with children. The Stationery Office, London
15. Department of Health 2001 Seeking consent: working with older people. The Stationery Office, London

16. Department of Health 2001 Seeking consent: working with people with learning disabilities. The Stationery Office, London
17. Department of Health 2001 Consent – what you have a right to expect [leaflets for patients, with versions for adults, children/young people, people with learning disabilities, parents and relatives/carers]. The Stationery Office, London
18. NHS Executive 2001 Good practice in consent: achieving the NHS plan commitment to patient-centred consent practice. Health Service Circular 2001/023
19. Department of Health 2001 Good practice in consent implementation [contains model policy and forms]. The Stationery Office, London
20. http://www.doh.gov.uk/tissue
21. Re C (adult: refusal of medical treatment) [1994] 1 WLR 290
22. Blundell C 1998 Competence in healthcare. In Wilson J, Tingle J (eds) Clinical risk modification, a route to clinical governance? Butterworth-Heinemann, Oxford
23. Re T (adult: refusal of consent) [1993] Fam Law 27
24. Gillick v West Norfolk Area Health Authority [1985] 3 AII ER 402
25. Airedale NHS Trust v Bland [1993] 4 Med LR 39
26. British Medical Journal 1999 Withholding and withdrawing life-prolonging medical treatment: guidance for decision making. BMJ Books, London
27. Ms B v An NHS Hospital Trust [2002] EWHC 429 (Fam)
28. Mental Health Act 1983, section 1(2)
29. Re F West Berkshire Health Authority [1989] 2 All ER 545
30. NHS Executive 2000 Resuscitation policy. Health Service Circular 2000/028
31. British Medical Association, Resuscitation Council (UK) and Royal College of Nursing [joint statement] 2001 Decisions relating to cardiopulmonary resuscitation http://www.resus.org.uk/pages/dnar.htm

Appendix 1
Clinical governance toolkit

Contents

1. Quality audit: a checklist for clinical governance. British Association of Medical Managers, 1998
2. Success criteria in clinical governance. NHS Executive, London Region, 1999
3. Silagy C, Mant D, Fowler G, Lodge M. Meta-analysis of efficacy of nicotine replacement therapies in smoking cessation. Lancet 1994; 343:139-42
4. Questions to assist with the critical appraisal of a systemic review (including at least one randomised controlled trial) (Type I evidence). University of Wales College of Medicine
5. Questions to assist with the critical appraisal of a randomised controlled trial) (Type II evidence). University of Wales College of Medicine
6. Questions to assist with the critical appraisal of an interventional study without randomisation (Type III evidence) or non experimental study (e.g. case control, cohort) (Type IV evidence). University of Wales College of Medicine
7. Questions to assist with the critical appraisal of a qualitative study (Type IV evidence). University of Wales College of Medicine
8. Questions to assist with the appraisal of an economic analysis paper
9. Appraisal instrument for clinical guidelines - version one. St George's Hospital Medical School, London, 1997
10. Appraisal of Guidelines for Research and Evaluation (AGREE) instrument. The AGREE Collaboration, www agreecollaboration.org, 2001
11. Planning a clinical audit - a checklist for good practice. National Centre for Clinical Audit (National Centre For Clinical Excellence), 1997

12. NCCA criteria for clinical audit. National Centre for Clinical Audit (National Centre For Clinical Excellence), 1997
13. Template annual report on clinical audit for a trust board. NHS Executive, London Region, 1999
14. Clinical negligence scheme for trusts – risk management standards – summary of standards and features. National Health Service Litigation Authority, 1999
15. Template annual report on risk management. NHS Executive, London Region, 1999

1. Quality audit: a checklist for clinical governance

Source: British Association of Medical Managers. Clinical Government: a document for consultation. 1998.

System	Process established?	Process explicit within organisation?	Process amenable to monitoring?	Reporting arrange-ments?	Implementation of findings/lessons monitored?	Levers & sanctions in place to make it work?
Quality improvement processes - clinical audit - integrated into organizational quality programme						
Leadership skills developed at clinical team level						
Evidence-based practice and infrastructure in place and used						
Clinical risk reduction programmes in place and of high quality						
Adverse events - detected, investigated, lessons learnt and translated into change in practice						
Systematic learning from clinical complaints, with translation into change in practice						
Poor clinical performance identified early and dealt with skill, speed and sensitivity, to avoid harm to patients						
Continuing professional development programmes in place, reflecting principles of clinical governance						
Quality of data for monitoring clinical care, of consistently high standard						

© BRITISH ASSOCIATION OF MEDICAL MANAGERS

2. Success criteria in clinical governance

Source: Discussion paper on success criteria in clinical governance, London Region website www.doh.gov.uk/ntro

SUCCESS CRITERION	MEANS OF VERIFICATION
CULTURE/ENVIRONMENT The organization has stated vision and values essential to 'Investment in People' processes Demonstrable use of well recognized quality management tools* Annual report presented to public demonstrating openness and public accountability **An agreed percentage in a proportion of staff who feel empowered to provide high quality care**	Report to board Documentary evidence Documentary evidence **Staff interviews**
STAFF AND ORGANIZATIONAL DEVELOPMENT An agreed percentage of professional staff with personal development plans (PDP) Clinical directors with job descriptions describing responsibilities for clinical quality and poorly performing staff Completed training programme for leaders Training programme for 'Investors in People' Training programme for each clinical directorate drawn up from the results of clinical audit, risk management and clinical effectiveness reviews Action plan to implement 'Maintaining Medical Excellence' is produced annually **Staff receive education and training relevant to their clinical practice**	Documentary evidence Documentary evidence Documentary evidence Documentary evidence Documentary evidence of outcome of PDP process Documentary evidence **Documentary of completion of training component of PDPs**
OVERALL GOVERNANCE An action plan incorporating issues in the BAMM checklist and a review of progress An annual report combining all sections presented to the board provides a critical assessment of progress **100 per cent of staff are involved in clinical governance**	Documentary evidence Documentary evidence **Staff interviews**
CLINICAL AUDIT The production of an annual audit report demonstrating comprehensive cover, appropriate selection, impact and value for money An increase in the proportion of audits using explicit standards from 30–60 per cent in 3 years An increase in the proportion of audits re-auditing and finding improved standards from 10–30 per cent in 3 years An agreed percentage increase in the proportion of all professional staff involved in at least one audit using the agreed standards resulting in an action plan devised by the clinical directorate and included in the business plan Each member of clinical staff is involved in audit An agreed percentage increase in the proportion of all multidisciplinary, multi-trust and externally verified audits and audits involving users and carers in the year **A mechanism in use (such as a clinical governance committee) to verify actions have taken place to rectify clinical audit findings with results documented** **Demonstrable changes to service organization or patient care as a result of audit**	Documentary evidence Analysis of audit projects using Oxford MAAG criteria Analysis of audit projects using Oxford MAAG criteria Documentary evidence Documentary evidence Documentary evidence **Reported in the annual audit report** **Reported in the annual audit report**

CLINICAL RISK MANAGEMENT Adoption of a blame-free policy espousing openness. A learning culture, facilitating critical self-examination of practice and finding ways to improve	Staff interviews
An increase in the number of clinical directorates with established risk management systems in place in high-risk specialties	Annual or quarterly report to board
A process of managing claims that minimizes stress to patients and staff	**Patient survey and staff interviews**
A risk management system with a single adverse event report producing an impact on patient care identified by a review of directorate action plans, an improved handling of complaints and a reduction in legal costs	**Annual report**
CLINICAL EFFECTIVENESS Specific training programme in critical appraisal skills for senior staff	Documentary evidence
The dissemination of latest evidence such as *Effectiveness Matters* and follow-up of appropriate action by directorate	Annual report
A system to digest national/NICE guidelines and implement them with an action plan for non-compliance	Annual report
Clinical policies and protocols scrutinized and approved by a policies committee that checks them against evidence	Documentary evidence
Increasing use of evidence-based medicine	**External audit****
Evidence of compliance with NICE and national service framework guidelines	**External audit**
QUALITY ASSURANCE An annual report bringing together a summary of all quality assurance work describing local standards, comparing performance with these standards and actions taken to improve the performance	Annual report
Complaints systematically analysed and documented action taken	Annual report
Benefits to patient care identified as a result of action following complaints investigation	Annual report
System in place to manage cross-directorate clinical quality, including the use, where appropriate of clinical pathways	Annual report
A complaints system that is open with patients, accepting fault where appropriate and providing a speedy response	**Patients survey**

* An example is the European Foundation for Quality Management (EFQM) model where:
- self assessment is a key part of the organization's performance management system
- staff at all levels are involved in the self-assessment process
- this provides a basis upon which plans for continuous improvements in the service is built.

** Ellis, J., Mulligan, I., Rowe, J. and Sackett, D. L. (1995). Inpatient general medicine is evidence based. *Lancet*, **346**, 407–410

NB: Process measures are in normal type and outcome measures are in bold type.

3. Meta-analysis

Meta-analysis on efficacy of nicotine replacement therapies in smoking cessation*

Christopher Silagy, David Mant, Godfrey Fowler, Mark Lodge

Summary

Nicotine-replacement therapy (NRT) by gum, transdermal patch, intranasal spray, or inhalation is expensive but how effective is it? We have done a meta-analysis of controlled trials to see how effects on abstinence rates are influenced by the clinical setting, the level of nicotine dependency, the dosage of NRT, and the intensity of additional advice and support offered. Published or unpublished randomised controlled trials of NRT that have assessed abstinence at least 6 months after the start of NRT were identified and 53 trials (42 gum, 9 patch, 1 intranasal spray, 1 inhaler), with data from 17 703 subjects, were included in the analyses.

Use of NRT increased the odds ratio (OR) of abstinence to 1·71 (95% confidence interval 1·56–1·87) compared with those allocated to the control interventions. The ORs for the different forms of NRT were 1·61 for gum, 2·07 for transdermal patch, 2·92 for nasal spray, and 3·05 for inhaled nicotine. These odds were non-significantly higher in subjects with higher levels of nicotine dependence but they were largely independent of the intensity of additional support provided or the setting in which NRT was offered.

We conclude that the currently available forms of NRT are effective therapies to aid smoking cessation.

Lancet 1994; **343:** 139–42

Introduction

Nicotine replacement is a frequent component of strategies to help people stop smoking.[1] The first type to become widely available was nicotine chewing gum but oral and gastric side-effects[2] impaired absorption when taken with coffee or acid beverages,[3] and a risk that some smokers might transfer their dependency to the gum[3] limited its usefulness. Other forms of nicotine replacement, devised to get round some of the problems with nicotine gum, are transdermal patches, intranasal sprays, and inhalers. Nicotine sprays and inhalers have not yet been licensed for general clinical use.

Systematic reviews of the efficacy of nicotine gum have been published.[1,4,5] In 1987, a meta-analysis of 14 trials concluded that the gum was most effective when used in

*Full version available electronically, with same authorship, under the title The Effectiveness of Nicotine Replacement Therapies in Smoking Cessation, as *Online Journal of Current Clinical Trials* 1994; 3: document no 113 (5 figures, 3 tables, 70 references).

Department of Public Health and Primary Care, University of Oxford, Radcliffe Infirmary, Oxford, UK (Prof C Silagy FRACGP, Prof D Mant MRCGP, G Fowler FRCGP, M Lodge)

Correspondence to: Prof Christopher Silagy, Department of General Practice, Flinders University of South Australia, School of Medicine, GPO Box 2100, Adelaide, South Australia 5001

specialised smoking cessation clinics and that it was of questionable value when used in general practice.[5] A 1990 review confirmed those findings.[1] However, since then there have been over 20 new randomised trials of nicotine gum. Two reviews of nicotine patches,[6,7] published in 1992, suggested that this form is also highly effective, but neither review used comprehensive methods to identify all the published and unpublished trials, nor did they use quantitative techniques to synthesise the data and test for homogeneity or significance.

Since nicotine replacement therapy is widely available and costly, it is important to establish the efficacy of its different forms when offered to smokers with varying levels of dependency and motivation to quit and to do so in a range of clinical settings, with or without additional support.[8] We have done a systematic review by meta-analysis of all randomised trials of nicotine gum, patches, sprays, and inhalers, in which participants have been followed up for at least 6 months.

Methods

Study selection

We did a computerised search with the DataStar program on seven databases to identify trials published before March, 1993. We also examined published reviews, reference lists from clinical trials, conference abstracts, smoking-and-health bulletins, and a bibliography on smoking and health. To identify unpublished studies we wrote to the manufacturers of nicotine replacement products.

To be included in the meta-analysis a trial had to have at least two treatment groups with allocation by formal randomisation or by a quasi-random method such as alternation. Studies with historical controls were excluded. The review was confined to a comparison of effects on smoking cessation rather than withdrawal symptoms. Trials in which follow-up was less than 6 months were also excluded. Side-effects were not reviewed quantitatively because of the wide variation in reporting the nature, timing, and duration of symptoms.

Definitions

Cessation rates were identified from the published reports and we used the strictest criterion to define abstinence, when there was a choice. Where biochemical confirmation of cessation was provided only those participants who met that criterion were regarded as being abstinent. Sustained cessation rates were used in preference to a point prevalence. Patients lost to follow-up were regarded as being continuing smokers. The methodological quality of the studies was also assessed.[9]

The intensity of additional support was defined as low if it could be regarded as routine care. If the time spent with the smoker (including assessment for the trial) exceeded 30 min at the first consultation or if the number of further assessment and reinforcement visits exceeded two, the intensity was classified as high.

Where the methodology was unclear or results were not expressed in a form which allowed extraction of key data we wrote to the investigators for the required information.

THE LANCET

NRT preparation	Proportion quitting		OR (95% CI)	χ¹ test for heterogeneity
	NRT	Control		
Gum (n = 39)	1149/6328 (18·2%)	893/8380 (10·6%)	1·61 (1·46–1·78)	$\chi^2_{38} = 49\cdot0, p = 0\cdot11$
Patches (n = 9)	255/1245 (20·5%)	105/968 (10·8%)	2·07 (1·64–2·62)	$\chi^2_8 = 7\cdot1, p = 0\cdot53$
Nasal spray (n = 1)	30/116 (25·9%)	11/111 (9·9%)	2·92 (1·49–5·74)	Not applicable
Inhaler (n = 1)	22/145 (15·2%)	7/141 (5·0%)	3·05 (1·42–6·57)	Not applicable
All NRT trials	1456/7834 (18·6%)	1016/9600 (10·6%)	1·71 (1·56–1·87)	$\chi^2_{44} = 64\cdot3, p = 0\cdot07$

Test for heterogeneity between different types of NRT ($\chi^2_3 = 8\cdot49, p = 0\cdot04$).
Based on longest follow-up available for each trial (minimum 6 months).

Table 1: **Comparison of proportion of smokers who successfully quit with NRT versus control**

Statistics

The statistical methods used to pool the data involved calculating the typical odds ratio (OR) and its 95% confidence interval (CI) on the basis of a fixed-effects model.[10] Heterogeneity was tested for by a Mantel-Haenszel approach.[11] Results are expressed as the OR (NRT to control) for achieving abstinence from smoking at a given time point together. The number of smokers that would have to be treated to produce one successful quitter at 12 months was derived from the inverse of the pooled typical event rate difference.[12] In subgroup analyses we used 12-month abstinence rates wherever possible, except for studies providing only 6 months of follow-up data.

Results

53 trials were included (42 gum, 9 patch, 1 spray, 1 inhaled).† Except for 12 gum trials and 3 patch trials, participants were followed up for at least 12 months. Only 1 trial restricted participation to male smokers.

31 gum trials used the 2 mg dose and 2 used 4 mg; 5 used a variable or mixed dosage; and in 4 trials the dose was not stated. The therapy lasted 3 weeks to 12 months. Many trials included dose tapering, but most encouraged participants to stop using the gum after 6–12 months. In the patch trials, the minimum duration of therapy ranged from 6 weeks to 3 months, with a tapering period, if required, in 3 studies.

The extent to which bias was controlled varied considerably. 39 trials made no attempt to describe randomisation; only 12 had blinded validation of smoking status of all those who reported abstinence. 21 trials reported the smoking status at the final follow-up visit of all participants randomised, including those who had withdrawn before the final assessment.

Despite great variation in trial characteristics there was no statistical evidence of significant heterogeneity. Only 3 trials yielded a negative treatment effect for nicotine replacement (OR < 1) at the end of follow-up, but in a further 31 trials the 95% CI included unity.

The four forms of nicotine replacement were all significantly more effective than placebo (or no therapy) in helping smokers to abstain. The benefit was evident throughout the 12 months of follow-up despite significant relapse rates. The odds of being abstinent at the four follow-up points during the 12 months remained fairly constant for each type of replacement.

When abstinence rates were pooled (table 1), according to the longest duration of follow-up available, 19% of those allocated to replacement and 11% of controls had successfully stopped smoking. This represents a 71% increase in the odds of abstinence with the use of nicotine replacement (95% CI 56–87%). On indirect comparison

the OR for abstinence with transdermal patches was greater than with nicotine gum, though this was not significant ($\chi^2_1 = 3\cdot69, p = 0\cdot05$). Similarly the ORs for abstinence with the newer forms of NRT (nasal spray and inhaler) were greater than with either nicotine gum or transdermal patch ($\chi^2_3 = 8\cdot49, p = 0\cdot04$). For trials of nicotine gum and transdermal patch, the odds of not smoking were not affected by whether the control group was placebo or no therapy (not shown).

The pooled odds of abstinence in the two trials which directly compared 4 mg with 2 mg gums was 76% greater with the higher dose (OR 1·76 [95% CI 0·99–3·13]). Only 1 trial compared a "fixed" dose regimen of nicotine gum with an "ad lib" regimen; the fixed dosage regimen increased the odds of abstinence but this was not significant (OR 1·36 [0·92–2·00]).

1 trial directly compared the effect of wearing nicotine patches only whilst awake (about 16 hours) versus

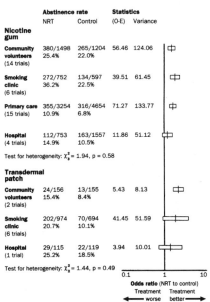

	Abstinence rate		Statistics		
	NRT	Control	(O-E)	Variance	
Nicotine gum					
Community volunteers (14 trials)	380/1498 25.4%	265/1204 22.0%	56.46	124.06	
Smoking clinic (6 trials)	272/752 36.2%	134/597 22.5%	39.51	61.45	
Primary care (15 trials)	355/3254 10.9%	316/4654 6.8%	71.27	133.77	
Hospital (4 trials)	112/753 14.9%	163/1557 10.5%	11.86	51.12	

Test for heterogeneity: $\chi^2_3 = 1.94, p = 0.58$

Transdermal patch					
Community volunteers (2 trials)	24/156 15.4%	13/155 8.4%	5.43	8.13	
Smoking clinic (6 trials)	202/974 20.7%	70/694 10.1%	41.45	51.59	
Hospital (1 trial)	29/115 25.2%	22/119 18.5%	3.94	10.01	

Test for heterogeneity: $\chi^2_2 = 1.44, p = 0.49$

Odds ratio (NRT to control)
Treatment worse — Treatment better

Figure: **Efficacy of nicotine gum and transdermal patches in different clinical settings**

Only pooled results for all trials within each subgroup shown. Graphical representation shows OR (vertical line) and 95% CI (box). Data are based on longest follow-up available for each study (minimum 6 months).

†A full list of trials is available from CS and appears in the *Online Journal of Current Clinical Trials* version of this paper.

THE LANCET

Setting	Intensity of support	Gum	Patch	Nasal spray	Inhaler
Any	Unselective	29 (22–41)	11 (8–18)		
Any	High	26 (17–58)	9 (6–20)	6 (4–16)	10 (6–30)
Any	Low	29 (21–45)	12 (8–30)		
Community volunteers	Unselective	15 (10–27)	10 (7–18)		
Smoking cessation clinics	Unselective	10 (7–19)		7 (4–16)	10 (6–30)
Primary care	Unselective	35 (25–63)	14 (7–222)		
Hospital patients	Unselective	58 (22–NE)	15 (6–NE)		

· · = no trials available.
NE = treatment not effective (ie, typical event difference favours control).
Data based only on trials which provided 12 month follow-up result.

Table 2: **Estimate of number of smokers needed to treat with NRT to produce one successful quitter at 12 months**

continuous wearing (24 hours). The study found no significant difference in the self-reported odds of abstinence at 6 months follow-up but had low power (OR for 24 h vs 16 h 0·62 [0·26–1·47]).

The efficacy of nicotine gum relative to control was similar whether offered to smokers attending smoking cessation clinics, to those recruited from the community as volunteers, or to patients recruited opportunistically through primary care (figure). However, since the absolute abstinence rate was higher in community volunteers and smoking cessation clinics, the percentage of smokers helped to quit by using NRT was higher in these settings than in primary care or hospital patients.

The proportional increase in the odds of smokers helped to quit by using transdermal patches is similar amongst those recruited either as community volunteers or opportunistically through primary care, although the 95% CIs for the ORs in primary care are wide, due to the small number of trials with 6–12 month follow-up data. Smokers recruited as hospital inpatients, or through outpatient clinics, have a non-significantly lower odds of quitting with either gum or transdermal patches than smokers seen in other clinical settings, and the confidence intervals even include unity. The nicotine gum results in this setting are also strongly influenced by one large trial which had a negative effect. The results for transdermal patches are based on small numbers of patients, since there is currently only one completed trial.

Four trials of 2 mg nicotine gum versus control stratified their results according to the smoker's level of nicotine dependence, assessed using the Fagerstrom score.[13] The OR for abstinence was not significantly greater in high nicotine dependent smokers with Fagerstrom scores $\geqslant 7$ (OR 2·48 [1·43–4·31] compared with 1·18 [0·70–2·01] in the low-dependency group with Fagerstrom scores < 7) ($\chi_1^2 = 3·61$, p = 0·06). Two trials compared 4 mg gum versus 2 mg gum in high nicotine-dependent smokers. The OR for abstinence was 2·7 (1·48–4·99) in favour of the 4 mg gum. Only one small trial compared 4 mg and 2 mg in smokers with low nicotine dependence; the results favouring the 2 mg dose (OR 0·27 [0·005–1·43]). There was insufficient data from the patch trials to stratify results according to the level of nicotine dependency.

To summarise the data from a clinical perspective we calculated the number of smokers who would require treatment with the various forms of NRT in order to produce 1 extra non-smoker at 12 months beyond the number who would achieve that with the control intervention (table 2).

The absolute probability of not smoking at 6–12 months was, not surprisingly, greater in trials which provided high-intensity additional support (19·7% [95% CI] 18·7–20·6%) rather than low intensity (10·5% [9·9–11·1%]). However, the OR for abstinence when nicotine gum was used in conjunction with low-intensity additional support (1·80 [1·54–2·11]) was not significantly different from the OR for abstinence when nicotine gum was used in conjunction with high-intensity support (1·48 [1·28–1·70]) ($\chi_1^2 = 3·39$, p = 0·07). Use of transdermal patches resulted in ORs of 2·14 (1·46–3·13) and 2·04 (1·51–2·74) with low and high intensity additional support, respectively; these ORs were not significantly different ($\chi_1^2 = 0·04$, p = 0·49). Only 2 small trials, both in primary care, directly compared the effect of providing high or low intensity follow-up to subjects receiving nicotine gum. The pooled results favour intensive follow-up but the result was not statistically significant (OR 1·30 [0·75–2·28).

Discussion

This overview provides reliable evidence, from nearly 18 000 subjects, that offering NRT to smokers, either as the mainstay of a smoking cessation strategy or as an adjunct to other interventions, is more effective in helping them to stop smoking than when NRT is not offered or if placebo is used. This applies to all forms of NRT and is independent of any variations in methodology or design characteristics of trials included in the overview.

All forms of NRT were associated with a high relapse rate. Minimising this relapse is important if long-term smoking cessation rates are to be substantially improved. Although considerable caution is required in drawing conclusions from indirect comparisons of efficacy both the absolute abstinence rate and the odds of abstinence were non-significantly greater with transdermal patches than nicotine gum. In clinical terms, our best estimate is that the number of smokers who would need to be "treated" could be reduced by up to 60% by using transdermal patches rather than nicotine gum. Two newer forms of NRT also show considerable promise although further trials are required. In addition, trials are required which directly compare the different types of NRT.

The two factors which have been suggested as the major determinants of the effectiveness of NRT are the setting in which it is offered and the smoker's level of dependency on nicotine.[15] The nature and flexibility of the dosage regimen seem far less important.

In this review the OR for abstinence with nicotine gum and transdermal patches was slightly greater if offered to smokers recruited from the community or those attending specialised clinics than if offered to smokers in primary care. However, these differences were not significant. Even if they had been, the number of specialised clinics will always be small so that access will be restricted to a small proportion of smokers wanting help to quit. The poor result seen with use of nicotine gum in hospital-based patients was disappointing given that these patients frequently had coexisting smoking-related diseases which might have been an added incentive to quit.

The benefit seen in previous studies of nicotine gum in smokers with high levels of dependency in nicotine is supported by the findings in this review although the difference in the ORs in the groups just failed to reach statistical significance. Further data from patch trials is required where abstinence rates are stratified according to the level of nicotine dependency.

THE LANCET

Addition of a high, rather than low, intensity support programme only reduced the number of smokers who needed to be treated with nicotine gum to produce 1 extra non-smoker at 12 moths from 29 to 26. For transdermal patches, the corresponding figures are 12 and 9, respectively. Smokers must not interpret these results as indicating that NRT offers an easy option "medical cure" for the far more complex problem of addictive behaviour. All the trials in this review included some form of support additional to NRT and it would be incorrect to conclude that such additional support is not necessary.

We thank the trialists who cooperated with our requests for clarification of previously reported data, ICRF Library Services for assistance in obtaining articles, Z Ilic and L Silagy for assistance with translations, and P Yudkin for statistical advice. CS is funded by the Sir Robert Menzies Memorial Trust and DM and ML are funded by the Imperial Cancer Research Fund.

References

1   Gourlay SG, McNeil JJ. Antismoking products. *Med J Aust* 1990; **153:** 699–707.

2   Henningfield JE, Radzius A, Cooper TM, Clayton RR. Drinking coffee and carbonated beverages blocks absorption of nicotine from nicotine polacrilex gum. *JAMA* 1990; **264:** 1560–64.

3   Hughes JR, Hatsukami DK, Skoog KP. Physical dependence on nicotine in gum. *JAMA* 1986; **255:** 3277–79.

4   Raw M. Does nicotine chewing gum work? *BMJ* 1985; **290:** 1231–32.

5   Lam W, Sze PC, Sacks HS, Chalmers TC. Meta-analysis of randomised controlled trials of nicotine chewing-gum. *Lancet* 1987; ii: 27–30.

6   Fiore MC, Jonerby DE, Baker TB, Kenford SL. Tobacco dependence and the nicotine patch. *JAMA* 1992; **268:** 2687–94.

7   Palmer KJ, Buckley MM, Faulds D. Transdermal nicotine: a review of its pharmacodynamic and pharmacokinetic properties, and therapeutic efficacy as an aid to smoking cessation. *Drugs* 1992; **44:** 498–529.

8   Saul H. Chancing your arm on nicotine patches. *New Sci* 1993; **137:** 12–13.

9   Chalmers I, Enkin M, Keirse MJNC, eds. Effective care in pregnancy and childbirth. Oxford: Oxford University Press, 1985.

10 Yusuf S, Peto R, Lewis J, Collins R, Sleight P. Beta-blockade during and after myocardial infarction: an overview of the randomised trials. *Prog Cardiovasc Dis* 1985; **27:** 335–71.

11 Cochran WG. The combination of estimates from different experiments. *Biometrics* 1954; **10:** 101–29.

12 Rothman KJ. Modern epidemiology. Boston: Little Brown, 1986: 186.

13 Fagerstrom KO. Measuring the degree of physical dependence to tobacco smoking with reference to individualization of treatment. *Addict Behav* 1978; **3:** 235–41.

4. Questions to assist with the critical appraisal of a systemic review (including at least one randomized controlled trial) – Type I evidence

Paper details   Authors:
                     Title:
                     Source:

A. What is this review about and can I trust it?   **Screening questions**

	Yes	Can't tell	No
1. Was the review conducted by a Cochrane Review Group, NHS Centre for Reviews & Dissemination, NHS Outcomes Agency or the Agency for Health Care Policy and Research (AHCPR)?	Go to question 8		Continue
2. Did the review address a clearly focused issue? In terms of: • the population studied • the intervention given • the outcomes considered			
3. Did the authors look for the appropriate sort of papers? Did the studies address the review's question and have an appropriate study design?			

Is it worth continuing?

Detailed questions

	Yes	Can't tell	No
4. Were the important relevant studies included? • Databases searched, reference list follow-up • Personal contacts, unpublished work • Non-English publications • Are the inclusion, exclusion criteria stated?			
5. Did the authors address the quality (rigour) of the included studies?			
6. If the results of the review have been combined, was this reasonable? • Were the studies sufficiently similar in design and results? • Are the results of included studies clearly displayed? • Are the reasons for any variation in the results discussed?			

B. What did they find?

7. What is the overall result of the review?	
Include a **numerical result** with the **confidence limits** if available	

C. Are the results relevant locally/to me?

	Yes	Can't tell	No
8. Can the results be applied to the local population? • Cultural differences? • Genetic differences? • Differences in medical practice?			
9. Were all important outcomes considered?			
10. Is any information provided which could help you decide whether the benefits are worth the harms/costs (financial and otherwise)? Summarize the cost information below, if available:		N/A	

From: Barker, J., Weightman, A. L. and Lancaster, J. (1997). Project for the enhancement of the Welsh protocols for investment in health gain. *Health Evidence Bulletins Wales, Project Methodology 2.* Department of Information Services, University of Wales College of Medicine.

5. Questions to assist with the critical appraisal of a randomized controlled trial – Type II evidence

Paper details   **Authors:**
                        Title:
                        Source:

A. What is this trial about and can I trust it?   **Screening questions**

	Yes	Can't tell	No
1. Did the trial address a clearly focused issue? In terms of: • the population studied • the intervention given • the outcomes considered			
2. Was the assignment of patients to treatments randomized?			
3. Were all the patients who entered the trial properly accounted for at its conclusion? • Was follow-up complete? • Were patients analysed in the groups to which they were randomized?			

Detailed questions

	Yes	Can't tell	No
4. Were patients, health workers and study personnel 'blind' to treatment? • Patients • Health workers • Study personnel			
5. Were the groups similar at the start of the trial? In terms of all the factors that might be relevant to the outcome: age, sex, social class, lifestyle etc.			
6. Aside from the experimental intervention, were the groups treated equally?			

Is it worth continuing?

B. What did they find?

7. How large was the treatment effect? • What outcomes were measured? • Take a note of the result(s) – e.g. odds ratio, numbers needed to treat, if provided	**Result(s):**
8. How precise was the estimate of the treatment effect? • What are the confidence limits? • Do you feel confident in the authors' use of statistics?	

C. Are the results relevant locally/to me?

	Yes	Can't tell	No
8. Can the results be applied to the local population? Do you think the patients covered by the trial are similar enough to your population? Consider culture, geography etc.			
9. Were all important outcomes considered? If not, does this affect the conclusion(s)?			
10. Is any information provided which could help you decide whether the benefits are worth the harms/costs (financial and otherwise)?			

From: Barker, J., Weightman, A. L. and Lancaster, J. (1997). Project for the enhancement of the Welsh protocols for investment in health gain. *Health Evidence Bulletins Wales, Project Methodology 2*. Department of Information Services, University of Wales College of Medicine.

6. Questions to assist with the critical appraisal of an interventional study without randomization – Type III evidence – or a non-experimental study (e.g. case-control, cohort) – Type IV evidence

Paper details **Authors:**
Title:
Source:

A. What is this paper about? **Screening questions**

	Yes	Can't tell	No
1. Did the paper address a clearly focused issue? Are the aims of the investigation clearly stated?			

B. Do I trust it?

	Yes	Can't tell	No
2. Have the authors reflected the current state of knowledge according to an unbiased review of the literature? • Has a sufficiently complete search of the relevant literature been carried out? • Is evidence included that is unfavourable to the authors' point of view?			
3. Is the choice of study method appropriate? • Has an acceptable method been chosen (e.g. interventional without randomization, case series, cross-sectional, cohort or case–control study)?[1] • Are the inclusion / exclusion criteria for patients given? • Is the choice of control group (if included) adequate?			

1. For an explanation of these study formats, see: Fowkes, F. G. R. and Fulton, P. M. (1991). Critical appraisal of published research: introductory guidelines. *Br. Med. J.*, **302**, 1136–40.

C. What did they find?

	Yes	Can't tell	No
4. Are tables/graphs adequately labelled and understandable?			
5. Are you confident with the authors' choice and use of statistical methods, if employed?			
6. What are the results of this piece of research? Are the authors' conclusions adequately supported by the information cited?			

D. Are the results relevant locally/to me?

	Yes	Can't tell	No
7. Can the results be applied to the local situation? Consider the differences between the local and study populations (e.g. cultural, geographical, ethical) which could affect the relevance of the study			
8. Were all important outcomes/results considered?			

From: Barker, J., Weightman, A. L. and Lancaster, J. (1997). Project for the enhancement of the Welsh protocols for investment in health gain. *Health Evidence Bulletins Wales, Project Methodology 2*. Department of Information Services, University of Wales College of Medicine.

7. Questions to assist with the critical appraisal of a qualitative study – Type IV evidence

Paper details   Authors:
               Title:
               Source:

A. What is this paper about?   **Screening questions**

	Yes	Can't tell	No
1. Did the paper address a clearly focused issue? Are the aims of the investigation clearly stated?			

B. Do I trust it?

	Yes	Can't tell	No
2. Is the choice of a qualitative approach appropriate? • What was this study exploring (e.g. behaviour/ reasoning/ beliefs)? • Do you think a quantitative approach could have equally/better addressed this issue?			
3. Was the author's position clearly stated? • Has the researcher described his/her perspective? • Has the researcher examined his/her role, potential bias and influence?			
4. Was the sampling strategy clearly described and justified? Check to see whether: • The method of sampling is stated or described • The investigators sampled the most useful or productive range of individuals and settings relevant to their question • The characteristics of those included in the study are defined			
5. Was there an adequate description of the method of data collection given? • Is the method of data collection described? • Is a rationale for the method given? • How was the data collected (e.g. audiotape/videotape/ field notes)? • Were appropriate data sources studied? • Were observations taken at different times?			

Section B continued	Yes	Can't tell	No
6. Were the procedures for data analysis/ interpretation described and justified? Check to see whether: • A description is given of how the themes and concepts were identified in the data • The analysis was performed by more than one researcher • Negative/discrepant results were taken into account • The data were fed back to the participants for comment			

C. What did they find?

	Yes	Can't tell	No
7. What are the primary findings? Consider whether the results: • Address the research question • Are likely to be clinically important			
8. Are the results credible? • Were sequences from original data presented (e.g. quotations?) • Is it possible to determine the source of the data presented (e.g. numbering of extracts)? • How much of the information collected is available for independent assessment? • Are the explanations for the results plausible and coherent? • Were external sources used to corroborate, elaborate or illuminate data (e.g. triangulation)?			

D. Are the results relevant locally?

	Yes	Can't tell	No
9. Can the results be applied to the local situation? • Consider the differences between the local and study populations (e.g. cultural, geographical, ethical) which could affect the relevance of the study • Have alternative explanations/theories for result been explored and discounted?			
10. Were all important outcomes/results considered?			

From: Barker, J., Weightman, A. L. and Lancaster, J. (1997). Project for the enhancement of the Welsh protocols for investment in health gain. *Health Evidence Bulletins Wales, Project Methodology 2*. Department of Information Services, University of Wales College of Medicine.

8. Questions to assist with the appraisal of an economic analysis paper

Paper details **Authors:**
               Title:
               Source:

A.   **What is this paper about?**

	Yes	Can't tell	No
1. Did the paper tackle a clearly defined clinical question about a subject that is economically important? (If the answer is no, do not proceed any further) Write down the reasons:			

B.   **Are the results of the paper valid?**

	Yes	Can't tell	No
2. Can you identify good evidence cited in the paper supporting the effectiveness of the interventions that are being compared?			
3. Is the method of economic analysis used appropriate for the intervention(s) studied?			
4. Are all the outcomes and costs identified, measured appropriately and valued?			
5. To test the robustness of the conclusions to the uncertainties in the data, did the authors perform a sensitivity analysis?			
Write down the reasons for the conclusions to this section			

C.   **What did they find?**

	Yes	Can't tell	No
6. Can you identify the following for each strategy? • The incremental costs • The absolute costs • The outcomes			
Summarise your findings			

D.   **Are the results relevant locally / to me?**

	Yes	Can't tell	No
7. Can the economic analysis be applied to the local situation/ my practice?			
8. Would the costs be similar in my setting?			
9. Do the benefits of treatment outweigh the harms and costs?			
Summarise your conclusions to this section			

Based on Drummond MF, Richardson WS, O'Brien BJ, and Levin M (1997). User's Guides to Medical Literature XIII. How to use an article on economic analysis of clinical practice. A. Are the results of the study valid? JAMA **277** xix 1552 - 7

9. Appraisal instrument for clinical guidelines – version 1

Appraisal Instrument
For Clinical Guidelines
Version One

Dimension 1: Rigour of Development

Responsibility for guideline development	Yes	No	Not sure	N/A	Notes
01 Is the agency responsible for the development of the guidelines clearly identified?					
02 Was external funding or other support received for developing the guidelines?					
03 If external funding or support was received, is there evidence that the potential biases of the funding body(ies) were taken into account?					

Guideline development group					
04 Is there a description of the individuals (e.g. professionals, interest groups – including patients) who were involved in the guidelines development group?					
05 If so, did the group contain representatives of all key disciplines?					

Identification and interpretation of evidence					
06 Is there a description of the sources of information used to select the evidence on which the recommendations are based?					
07 If so, are the sources of information adequate?					
08 Is there a description of the method(s) used to interpret and assess the strength of the evidence?					
09 If so, is(are) the method(s) for rating the evidence satisfactory?					

Formulation of recommendations					
10 Is there a description of the methods used to formulate the recommendations?					
11 If so, are the methods satisfactory?					
12 Is there an indication of how the views of interested parties not on the panel were taken into account?					

Appraisal Instrument
For Clinical Guidelines
Version One
Dimension 1: Rigour of Development

Formulation of recommendations (cont.)	Yes	No	Not sure	N/A	Notes
13 Is there an explicit link between the major recommendations and the level of supporting evidence?					

Peer review					
14 Were the guidelines independently reviewed prior to their publication/release?					
15 If so, is explicit information given about methods and how comments were addressed?					
16 Were the guidelines piloted?					
17 If the guidelines were piloted, is explicit information given about the methods used and the results adopted?					

Updating					
18 Is there a mention of a date for reviewing or updating the guidelines?					
19 Is the body responsible for the reviewing and updating clearly identified?					

Overall assessment of development process					
20 Overall, have the potential biases of guideline development been adequately dealt with?					

Further Comments:

Appraisal Instrument
For Clinical Guidelines
Version One # Dimension 2: Context and Content

Objectives	Yes	No	Not sure	N/A	Notes
21 Are the reasons for developing the guidelines clearly stated?					
22 Are the objectives of the guidelines clearly defined?					

Context					
23 Is there a satisfactory description of the patients to which the guidelines are meant to apply?					
24 Is there a description of the circumstances (clinical or non-clinical) in which exceptions might be made in using the guidelines?					
25 Is there an explicit statement of how patients' preferences should be taken into account in applying the guidelines?					

Clarity					
26 Do the guidelines describe the condition to be detected, treated, or prevented in unambiguous terms?					
27 Are the different possible options for management of the condition clearly stated in the guidelines?					
28 Are the recommendations clearly presented?					

Likely costs and benefits					
29 Is there an adequate description of the health benefits that are likely to be gained from the recommended management?					
30 Is there an adequate description of the potential harms or risks that may occur as a result of the recommended management?					
31 Is there an estimate of the costs or expenditures likely to incur from the recommended management?					
32 Are the recommendations supported by the estimated benefits, harms and costs of the intervention?					

Appraisal Instrument
For Clinical Guidelines
Version One
Dimension 3: Application

Guideline dissemination & implementation	Yes	No	Not sure	N/A	Notes
33 Does the guideline document suggest possible methods for dissemination and implementation?					

Monitoring of guidelines/clinical audit					
34 Does the guideline document specify criteria for monitoring compliance?					
35 Does the guideline document identify clear standards or targets?					
36 Does the guideline document define measurable outcomes that can be monitored?					

National guidelines only					
37 Does the guideline document identify key elements which need to be considered by local guideline groups?					

Further Comments:

10. Appraisal of guidelines for research and evaluation

The AGREE Collaboration
September 2001

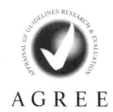

AGREE

INTRODUCTION

Purpose of the AGREE Instrument.

The purpose of the Appraisal of Guidelines Research & Evaluation (AGREE) Instrument is to provide a framework for assessing the quality of clinical practice guidelines.

Clinical practice guidelines are 'systematically developed statements to assist practitioner and patient decisions about appropriate health care for specific clinical circumstances'[1]. Their purpose is 'to make explicit recommendations with a definite intent to influence what clinicians do'[2].

By quality of clinical practice guidelines we mean the confidence that the potential biases of guideline development have been addressed adequately and that the recommendations are both internally and externally valid, and are feasible for practice. This process involves taking into account the benefits, harms and costs of the recommendations, as well as the practical issues attached to them. Therefore, the assessment includes judgements about the methods used for developing the guidelines, the content of the final recommendations, and the factors linked to their uptake.

The AGREE Instrument assesses both the quality of the reporting, and the quality of some aspects of recommendations. It provides an assessment of the predicted validity of a guideline, that is the likelihood that it will achieve its intended outcome. It does not assess the impact of a guideline on patients' outcomes.

Most of the criteria contained in the AGREE Instrument are based on theoretical assumptions rather than on empirical evidence. They have been developed through discussions between researchers from several countries who have extensive experience and knowledge of clinical guidelines. Thus, the AGREE Instrument should be perceived as reflecting the current state of knowledge in the field.

Which guidelines can be appraised with the AGREE Instrument.

The AGREE Instrument is designed to assess guidelines developed by local, regional, national or international groups or affiliated governmental organisations. These include:

1. New guidelines
2. Existing guidelines
3. Updates of existing guidelines

The AGREE Instrument is generic and can be applied to guidelines in any disease area including those for diagnosis, health promotion, treatment or interventions. It is suitable for guidelines presented in paper or electronic format.

[1] Lohr KN, Field MJ. A provisional instrument for assessing clinical practice guidelines. In: Field MJ, Lohr KN (eds). Guidelines for clinical practice. From development to use. Washington D.C. National Academy Press, 1992.

[2] Hayward RSA, Wilson MC, Tunis SR, Bass EB, Guyatt G, for the Evidence-Based Medicine Working Group. Users' guides to the Medical Literature. VIII. How to Use Clinical Practice Guidelines. A. Are the Recommendations Valid? JAMA, 1995;274, 570-574.

AGREE APPRAISAL INSTRUMENT

AGREE

INTRODUCTION

Who can use the AGREE Instrument?

The AGREE Instrument is intended to be used by the following groups:

i) By policy makers to help them decide which guidelines could be recommended for use in practice. In such instances, the instrument should be part of a formal assessment process.
ii) By guideline developers to follow a structured and rigorous development methodology and as a self-assessment tool to ensure that their guidelines are sound.
iii) By health care providers who wish to undertake their own assessment before adopting the recommendations
iv) By educators or teachers to help enhance critical appraisal skills amongst health professionals.

Key references

The following sources have been used for developing the AGREE Instrument criteria.

Lohr KN, Field MJ. A provisional instrument for assessing clinical practice guidelines. In: Field MJ, Lohr KN (eds). Guidelines for clinical practice. From development to use. Washington D.C. National Academy Press, 1992.

Cluzeau F, Littlejohns P, Grimshaw J, Feder G, Moran S. Development and application of a generic methodology to assess the quality of clinical guidelines. International Journal for Quality in Health Care 1999;11:21-28.

Grol R, Dalhuijzen J, Mokkink H, Thomas S, Veld C, Rutten G. Attributes of clinical guidelines that influence use of guidelines in general practice: observational study. BMJ 1998;317:858-861.

Lohr KN. The quality of practice guidelines and the quality of health care. In: Guidelines in health care. Report of a WHO Conference. January 1997, Baden-Baden: Nomos Verlagsgesellschaft, 1998.

AGREE APPRAISAL INSTRUMENT

INSTRUCTIONS FOR USE

Please read the following instructions carefully before using the AGREE Instrument.

1. Structure and content of the AGREE Instrument

AGREE consists of 23 key items organised in six domains. Each domain is intended to capture a separate dimension of guideline quality.

Scope and purpose (items 1-3) is concerned with the overall aim of the guideline, the specific clinical questions and the target patient population.

Stakeholder involvement (items 4-7) focuses on the extent to which the guideline represents the views of its intended users.

Rigour of development (items 8-14) relates to the process used to gather and synthesise the evidence, the methods to formulate the recommendations and to update them.

Clarity and presentation (items 15-18) deals with the language and format of the guideline.

Applicability (items 19-21) pertains to the likely organisational, behavioural and cost implications of applying the guideline.

Editorial independence (items 22-23) is concerned with the independence of the recommendations and acknowledgement of possible conflict of interest from the guideline development group.

2. Documentation

Appraisers should attempt to identify all information about the guideline development process prior to appraisal. This information may be contained in the same document as the recommendations or it may be summarised in a separate technical report, in published papers or in policy reports (e.g. guideline programmes). We recommend that you read the guideline and its accompanying documentation fully before you start the appraisal.

3. Number of appraisers

We recommend that each guideline is assessed by at least two appraisers and preferably four as this will increase the reliability of the assessment.

4. Response scale

Each item is rated on a 4-point scale ranging from 4 'Strongly Agree' to 1 'Strongly Disagree', with two mid points: 3 'Agree' and 2 'Disagree'. The scale measures the extent to which a criterion (item) has been fulfilled.

- If you are confident that the criterion has been fully met then you should answer 'Strongly Agree'.

- If you are confident that the criterion has not been fulfilled at all or if there is no information available then you should answer 'Strongly Disagree'.

- If you are unsure that a criterion has been fulfilled, for example because the information is unclear or because only some of the recommendations fulfil the criterion, then you should answer 'Agree' or 'Disagree', depending on the extent to which you think the issue has been addressed.

5. User Guide

We have provided additional information in the User Guide adjacent to each item. This information is intended to help you understand the issues and concepts addressed by the item. Please read this guidance carefully before giving your response.

AGREE APPRAISAL INSTRUMENT

INSTRUCTIONS FOR USE

AGREE

Please read the following instructions carefully before using the AGREE Instrument.

6. Comments
There is a box for comments next to each item. You should use this box to explain the reasons for your responses. For example, you may 'Strongly Disagree' because the information is not available, the item is not applicable, or the methodology described in the information provided is unsatisfactory. Space for further comments is provided at the end of the instrument.

7. Calculating domain scores
Domain scores can be calculated by summing up all the scores of the individual items in a domain and by standardising the total as a percentage of the maximum possible score for that domain.

Example:

If four appraisers give the following scores for Domain 1 (Scope & purpose):

	Item 1	Item 2	Item 3	Total
Appraiser 1	2	3	3	8
Appraiser 2	3	3	4	10
Appraiser 3	2	4	3	9
Appraiser 4	2	3	4	9
Total	**9**	**13**	**14**	**36**

Maximum possible score = 4 (strongly agree) x 3 (items) x 4 (appraisers) = 48
Minimum possible score = 1 (strongly disagree) x 3 (items) x 4 (appraisers) = 12

The standardised domain score will be:

$$\frac{\text{obtained score} - \text{minimum possible score}}{\text{Maximum possible score} - \text{minimum possible score}} =$$

$$\frac{36-12}{48-12} = \frac{24}{36} = 0.67 \times 100 = 67\%$$

Note:
The six domain scores are independent and should not be aggregated into a single quality score. Although the domain scores may be useful for comparing guidelines and will inform the decision as to whether or not to use or to recommend a guideline, it is not possible to set thresholds for the domain scores to mark a 'good' or 'bad' guideline.

8. Overall assessment
A section for overall assessment is included at the end of the instrument. This contains a series of options 'Strongly recommend', 'Recommend (with provisos or alterations)', 'Would not recommend' and 'Unsure'. The overall assessment requires the appraiser to make a judgement as to the quality of the guideline, taking each of the appraisal criteria into account.

AGREE APPRAISAL INSTRUMENT

SCOPE AND PURPOSE

1. The overall objective(s) of the guideline is (are) specifically described.

Strongly Agree	4	3	2	1	Strongly Disagree

Comments

2. The clinical question(s) covered by the guideline is(are) specifically described.

Strongly Agree	4	3	2	1	Strongly Disagree

Comments

3. The patients to whom the guideline is meant to apply are specifically described.

Strongly Agree	4	3	2	1	Strongly Disagree

Comments

USER GUIDE

SCOPE AND PURPOSE

AGREE

1.

This deals with the potential health impact of a guideline on society and populations of patients. The overall objective(s) of the guideline should be described in detail and the expected health benefits from the guideline should be specific to the clinical problem. For example specific statements would be:
- Preventing (long term) complications of patients with diabetes mellitus;
- Lowering the risk of subsequent vascular events in patients with previous myocardial infarction;
- Rational prescribing of antidepressants in a cost-effective way.

2.

A detailed description of the clinical questions covered by the guideline should be provided, particularly for the key recommendations (see item 17). Following the examples provided in question 1:
- How many times a year should the HbA1c be measured in patients with diabetes mellitus?
- What should the daily aspirin dosage for patients with proven acute myocardial infarction be?
- Are selective serotonin reuptake inhibitors (SSRIs) more cost-effective than tricyclic antidepressants (TCAs) in treatment of patients with depression?

3.

There should be a clear description of the target population to be covered by a guideline. The age range, sex, clinical description, comorbidity may be provided. For example:
- A guideline on the management of diabetes mellitus only includes patients with non-insulin dependent diabetes mellitus and excludes patients with cardiovascular comorbidity.
- A guideline on the management of depression only includes patients with major depression, according to the DSM-IV criteria, and excludes patients with psychotic symptoms and children.
- A guideline on screening of breast cancer only includes women, aged between 50 and 70 years, with no history of cancer and with no family history of breast cancer.

AGREE APPRAISAL INSTRUMENT

STAKEHOLDER INVOLVEMENT

4. The guideline development group includes individuals from all the relevant professional groups.

| Strongly Agree | 4 | 3 | 2 | 1 | Strongly Disagree |

Comments

5. The patients' views and preferences have been sought.

| Strongly Agree | 4 | 3 | 2 | 1 | Strongly Disagree |

Comments

6. The target users of the guideline are clearly defined.

| Strongly Agree | 4 | 3 | 2 | 1 | Strongly Disagree |

Comments

7. The guideline has been piloted among target users.

| Strongly Agree | 4 | 3 | 2 | 1 | Strongly Disagree |

Comments

USER GUIDE

STAKEHOLDER INVOLVEMENT

A G R E E

4.

This item refers to the professionals who were involved at some stage of the development process. This may include members of the steering group, the research team involved in selecting and reviewing/rating the evidence and individuals involved in formulating the final recommendations. This item excludes individuals who have externally reviewed the guideline (see Item 13). Information about the composition, discipline and relevant expertise of the guideline development group should be provided.

5.

Information about patients' experiences and expectations of health care should inform the development of clinical guidelines. There are various methods for ensuring that patients' perspectives inform guideline development. For example, the development group could involve patients' representatives, information could be obtained from patient interviews, literature reviews of patients' experiences could be considered by the group. There should be evidence that this process has taken place.

6.

The target users should be clearly defined in the guideline, so they can immediately determine if the guideline is relevant to them. For example, the target users for a guideline on low back pain may include general practitioners, neurologists, orthopaedic surgeons, rheumatologists and physiotherapists.

7.

A guideline should have been pre-tested for further validation amongst its intended end users prior to publication. For example, a guideline may have been piloted in one or several primary care practices or hospitals. This process should be documented.

AGREE APPRAISAL INSTRUMENT

RIGOUR OF DEVELOPMENT

8. Systematic methods were used to search for evidence.

Strongly Agree	4	3	2	1	Strongly Disagree

Comments

9. The criteria for selecting the evidence are clearly described.

Strongly Agree	4	3	2	1	Strongly Disagree

Comments

10. The methods used for formulating the recommendations are clearly described.

Strongly Agree	4	3	2	1	Strongly Disagree

Comments

11. The health benefits, side effects and risks have been considered in formulating the recommendations.

Strongly Agree	4	3	2	1	Strongly Disagree

Comments

USER GUIDE

RIGOUR OF DEVELOPMENT

A G R E E

8.

Details of the strategy used to search for evidence should be provided including search terms used, sources consulted and dates of the literature covered. Sources may include electronic databases (e.g. MEDLINE, EMBASE, CINAHL), databases of systematic reviews (e.g. the Cochrane Library, DARE), handsearching journals, reviewing conference proceedings and other guidelines (e.g. the US National Guideline Clearinghouse, the German Guidelines Clearinghouse).

9.

Criteria for including/excluding evidence identified by the search should be provided. These criteria should be explicitly described and reasons for including and excluding evidence should be clearly stated. For example, guideline authors may decide to only include evidence from randomised clinical trials and to exclude articles not written in English.

10.

There should be a description of the methods used to formulate the recommendations and how final decisions were arrived at. Methods include for example, a voting system, formal consensus techniques (e.g. Delphi, Glaser techniques). Areas of disagreement and methods of resolving them should be specified.

11.

The guideline should consider health benefits, side effects, and risks of the recommendations. For example, a guideline on the management of breast cancer may include a discussion on the overall effects on various final outcomes. These may include: survival, quality of life, adverse effects, and symptom management or a discussion comparing one treatment option to another. There should be evidence that these issues have been addressed.

AGREE APPRAISAL INSTRUMENT

RIGOUR OF DEVELOPMENT

12. There is an explicit link between the recommendations and the supporting evidence.

Strongly Agree	4	3	2	1	Strongly Disagree

Comments

13. The guideline has been externally reviewed by experts prior to its publication.

Strongly Agree	4	3	2	1	Strongly Disagree

Comments

14. A procedure for updating the guideline is provided.

Strongly Agree	4	3	2	1	Strongly Disagree

Comments

AGREE

RIGOUR OF DEVELOPMENT

12.

There should be an explicit link between the recommendations and the evidence on which they are based. Each recommendation should be linked with a list of references on which it is based.

13.

A guideline should be reviewed externally before it is published. Reviewers should not have been involved in the development group and should include some experts in the clinical area and some methodological experts. Patients' representatives may also be included. A description of the methodology used to conduct the external review should be presented, which may include a list of the reviewers and their affiliation.

14.

Guidelines need to reflect current research. There should be a clear statement about the procedure for updating the guideline. For example, a timescale has been given, or a standing panel receives regularly updated literature searches and makes changes as required.

AGREE APPRAISAL INSTRUMENT

CLARITY AND PRESENTATION

15. The recommendations are specific and unambiguous.

Strongly Agree	4	3	2	1	Strongly Disagree

Comments

16. The different options for management of the condition are clearly presented.

Strongly Agree	4	3	2	1	Strongly Disagree

Comments

17. Key recommendations are easily identifiable.

Strongly Agree	4	3	2	1	Strongly Disagree

Comments

18. The guideline is supported with tools for application.

Strongly Agree	4	3	2	1	Strongly Disagree

Comments

USER GUIDE

CLARITY AND PRESENTATION

AGREE

15.

A recommendation should provide a concrete and precise description of which management is appropriate in which situation and in what patient group, as permitted by the body of evidence.
- An example of a specific recommendation is: Antibiotics have to be prescribed in children of two years or older with acute otitis media if the complaint last longer than three days or if the complaint increase after the consultation despite adequate treatment with painkillers; in these cases amoxycillin should be given for 7 days (supplied with a dosage scheme).
- An example of a vague recommendation is: Antibiotics are indicated for cases with an abnormal or complicated course.

However, evidence is not always clear cut and there may be uncertainty about the best management. In this case the uncertainty should be stated in the guideline.

16.

A guideline should consider the different possible options for screening, prevention, diagnosis or treatment of the condition it covers. These possible options should be clearly presented in the guideline. For example, a recommendation on the management of depression may contain the following alternatives:
  a. Treatment with TCA
  b. Treatment with SSRI
  c. Psychotherapy
  d. Combination of pharmacological and psychological therapy

17.

Users should be able to find the most relevant recommendations easily. These recommendations answer the main clinical questions that have been covered by the guideline. They can be identified in different ways. For example, they can be summarised in a box, typed in bold, underlined or presented as flow charts or algorithms.

18.

For a guideline to be effective it needs to be disseminated and implemented with additional materials. These may include for example, a summary document, or a quick reference guide, educational tools, patients' leaflets, computer support, and should be provided with the guideline.

15

AGREE APPRAISAL INSTRUMENT

APPLICABILITY

---

19. The potential organisational barriers in applying the recommendations have been discussed.

| Strongly Agree | 4 | 3 | 2 | 1 | Strongly Disagree |

Comments

---

20. The potential cost implications of applying the recommendations have been considered.

| Strongly Agree | 4 | 3 | 2 | 1 | Strongly Disagree |

Comments

---

21. The guideline presents key review criteria for monitoring and/or audit purposes.

| Strongly Agree | 4 | 3 | 2 | 1 | Strongly Disagree |

Comments

16

APPLICABILITY

A G R E E

19.

Applying the recommendations may require changes in the current organisation of care within a service or a clinic which may be a barrier to using them in daily practice. Organisational changes that may be needed in order to apply the recommendations should be discussed. For example:
  i. A guideline on stroke may recommend that care should be co-ordinated through stroke units and stroke services.
  ii. A guideline on diabetes in primary care may require that patients are seen and followed up in diabetic clinics.

20.

The recommendations may require additional resources in order to be applied. For example, there may be a need for more specialised staff, new equipment, expensive drug treatment. These may have cost implications for health care budgets. There should be a discussion of the potential impact on resources in the guideline.

21.

Measuring the adherence to a guideline can enhance its use. This requires clearly defined review criteria that are derived from the key recommendations in the guideline. These should be presented. Examples of review criteria are:
• The HbA1c should be < 8.0%.
• The level of diastolic blood pressure should be < 95 mmHg.
• If complaints of acute otitis media lasts longer than three days amoxicillin should be prescribed.

AGREE APPRAISAL INSTRUMENT

EDITORIAL INDEPENDENCE

22. The guideline is editorially independent from the funding body.

Strongly Agree	4	3	2	1	Strongly Disagree

Comments

23. Conflicts of interest of guideline development members have been recorded.

Strongly Agree	4	3	2	1	Strongly Disagree

Comments

FURTHER COMMENTS

EDITORIAL INDEPENDENCE

AGREE

22.

Some guidelines are developed with external funding (e.g. Government funding, charity organisations, pharmaceutical companies). Support may be in the form of financial contribution for the whole development, or for parts of it, e.g. printing of the guidelines. There should be an explicit statement that the views or interests of the funding body have not influenced the final recommendations. Please note: If it is stated that a guideline was developed without external funding, then you should answer 'Strongly Agree'.

23.

There are circumstances when members of the development group may have conflicts of interest. For example, this would apply to a member of the development group whose research on the topic covered by the guideline is also funded by a pharmaceutical company. There should be an explicit statement that all group members have declared whether they have any conflict of interest.

FURTHER COMMENTS

11. Planning a clinical audit

NB: NCCA is now absorbed into NICE

National Centre for Clinical Audit
Information for better healthcare

The National Centre for Clinical Audit
90 Long Acre
Covent Garden
London WC2E 9RZ

PLANNING A CLINICAL AUDIT – A CHECKLIST FOR GOOD PRACTICE

As you and/or your colleagues plan a specific audit, work through this checklist to help you consider how you will carry out each step in the process.

DESIGN

1. Involve Stakeholders

Which of the following individuals or groups should be involved in designing the audit: (*Tick all that apply.*)

❑ Clinical or other staff involved in delivering the care or service in this organization
❑ Clinical or other staff involved in delivering the care or service in (an)other organization(s)
❑ People who receive the care or use the service
❑ People who may be involved in any changes in practice that the audit might show are needed

How should each individual or group be involved? (*Tick all that apply. Who should be involved?*)

❑ Participate in designing the audit ....
❑ Consult on the design of the audit ....
❑ Provide information for the audit ....
❑ Receive feedback about the audit later ....
❑ Participate in planning or carrying out action ....

2. Select an Important Topic

Which of the following reflects why the topic was selected. (*Tick all that apply.*)

❑ Findings of a systematic review of the literature
❑ Affects a large number of patients, clients, or users
❑ Involves higher than usual risk to patients, staff, or the organization
❑ Is a concern about quality raised by staff, patients, relatives, purchasers, or managers
❑ Has potential for improving the effectiveness of care or service
❑ The intervention or service is costly or there is potential to improve cost effectiveness
❑ Other, e.g. purchaser priority ....
....

3. **State Objectives**

Do the objectives for the audit reflect both of the following:

❏ The reason the audit is being carried out *and*
❏ What the group intends to achieve through the audit

4. **Use Explicit Measures**

Are there explicit measures of quality care or service or of good practice to use in the audit from either of the following:

❏ Available from literature, a professional or other organization, or other source *and/or*
❏ Developed by the audit group

5. **Reflect Good Practice**

Are the audit objectives and the measures being used in the audit consistent with all of the following?

❏ Reflect the best available evidence of good practice *and*
❏ Are acceptable to the practitioners whose care will be assessed *and*
❏ Do not involve collecting information on outcome only

6. **Define Case Selection**

Are *all* of the following defined?

❏ The nature of what is to be audited — cases, episodes, events, situations, circumstances, letters, etc.
❏ The number of cases to be included in the audit
❏ The types of cases which are to be included or excluded
❏ How the specific cases are to be identified and how records or other data sources are to be located
❏ The time period from which cases are to be drawn
❏ Any cases which are excluded after data collection begins — and the reason why the cases were excluded

Are the cases to be included in the audit and how they are selected:

❏ Appropriate for the audit objectives *and*
❏ Appropriate for the measures being used in the audit

MEASURE

7. **Test Validity and Reliability of Data**

Do the data to be collected for the audit:

❏ Relate directly to the objectives *and*
❏ Relate directly to the measures being used in the audit

Does the description of data to be collected for the audit:

❏ Include definitions and synonyms of key terms, acceptable abbreviations, numeric values or ranges of values, including times as appropriate *and*
❏ Include instructions for where to find the information

8. **Respect Ethics and Confidentiality**

Do data collection procedures and forms meet:

❑ Accepted ethical principles **and**
❑ Agreed confidentiality policies

9. **Analyse Audit Data**

Are data grouped and analysed to achieve **all** of the following?

❑ Give a complete, accurate, and unbiased view of actual practice **and**
❑ Relate directly to the audit objectives and measures **and**
❑ Identify useful information for the audit group

EVALUATE

10. **Present Audit Data**

Are data presented to include the following:

❑ Cases which are determined in advance to be *clinically acceptable* exceptions as meeting the agreed audit measures **and**
❑ Cases which are determined through structured peer review to be *clinically acceptable* exceptions as meeting the agreed audit measures

Are data presented to help the audit group to see the following:

❑ The degree to which actual practice is consistent with good practice **and**
❑ Any shortcomings in actual practice.

11. **Identify Shortcomings and their Causes**

Based on evaluation and analysis of the audit findings, does the audit group identify:

❑ Any specific shortcomings in actual care **and**
❑ Causes of these shortcomings

12. **Identify Needed Improvements**

Does the audit group identify:

❑ The specific improvements in practice which are needed, if any **and**
❑ What making the improvements will involve

ACT

13. Devise a Strategy for Action

Does the audit group consider *all* of the following:

- ☐ What exactly has to change
- ☐ If there is a readiness to change
- ☐ What the most likely way is to achieve change and what are alternative ways
- ☐ How the steps will be taken to implement the change
- ☐ Who needs to act and to or for whom
- ☐ When the action will take place
- ☐ How and when the group will know if things are going according to plan
- ☐ How the group will know if the action taken actually worked

14. Implement Action

Does the audit group assume responsibility for the following:

- ☐ Implementing the action plan *and/or*
- ☐ Referring to others the need for action and a suggested realistic plan for actions which are outside the control of the group *and*
- ☐ Providing feedback to stakeholders, at least concerning any actions planned or taken

Is evidence available to:

- ☐ Confirm that audit findings have been acted upon *and/or*
- ☐ Support reasons for lack of action when action is not taken

REPEAT FOR IMPROVEMENT

15. Repeat the Process

Is the audit process repeated (i.e. reaudit is carried out) in the following circumstances:

- ☐ Needed improvements are not yet achieved at the required or target level
  (unless despite repeated best efforts to improve practice, due to circumstances outside the control of the audit group, performance is unlikely to improve further and those responsible have been informed of actions taken and reaudit findings) *or*
- ☐ Circumstances in the provision of care or service related to the audit topic have changed significantly in ways which may negatively affect the quality of care or service, e.g. the service has been relocated, or there is a major turnover of staff who provide the service

Contact your local clinical audit department, your Primary Care Audit Group or Medical Audit Advisory Group, your professional organization, or the NCCA for more information on the NCCA Criteria for Clinical Audit.

12. NCCA criteria for clinical audit

NB: NCCA is now absorbed into NICE

National Centre for Clinical Audit
Information for better healthcare

The National Centre for Clinical Audit
90 Long Acre
Covent Garden
London WC2E 9RZ

NCCA CRITERIA FOR CLINICAL AUDIT

The purpose of the NCCA Criteria for Clinical Audit is to provide guidance on good practice in clinical audit for practitioners carrying out clinical audits, local or national audit groups or committees, purchasers funding audit programmes, and others.

		CRITERION	EXPLANATION
DESIGN	1	Stakeholders in a service contribute ideas for audits and are involved in the audit process as appropriate.	Patients or clients, carers, internal or external service users, and purchasers, as appropriate, are enabled to suggest topics for audit, directly or indirectly, to the individual or group responsible for audit in a service. Stakeholders also may suggest aspects of the quality of care or service to be included in an audit and may participate in the audit process, as appropriate.
	2	The topics selected for audit are important to the quality of care.	Important topics are those which involve one or more of the following: • A large number of patients or clients. • Higher than usual risk to patients or staff. • A concern about the quality of care raised by patients, carers, users, staff, or purchasers. • Potential for improving the effectiveness of care or service. • A costly intervention or service or the potential to improve cost effectiveness.
	3	One or more specific quality improvement-related objectives for an audit are stated.	Objectives are defined clearly and are foxused on achieving improvement in the quality of care or service. Objectives consider stakeholders' views as far as possible.
	4	Explicit measures of one or more aspects of quality of care or service are established to enable comparison between actual practice and good practice.	Explicit measures state clearly and unambiguously what is to be assessed about actual practice. They can be about any aspect of care or service that is relevant to the audit objectives, including: documentation or information; critical processes; clinical, educational, or behavioural outcomes; critical incidents; or adverse events.
	5	The audit objectives and measures reflect the best available evidence of good practice.	The audit design reflects up-to-date, sound evidence of good practice. If research evidence is not available for a topic, the audit design reflects national or local consensus on good practice.
	6	The number and type of cases to be included in an audit, and the time period over which they are to be drawn, are defined clearly and are appropriate to the audit objectives and measures.	The number of cases, episodes, or occurrences and how they are to be selected, including any to be excluded, are described **before** data are collected. If cases are identified for inclusion in an audit but are excluded subsequently, the reason is stated clearly.

		CRITERION	EXPLANATION
MEASURE	7	Valid and reliable data are collected to enable a comparison between actual practice and good practice.	Audit data are valid if they relate directly to the agreed objectives and measures. Audit data are reliable if different people collecting data, or the same person collecting the same data at different times, make(s) the same or almost the same judgements about actual practice.
	8	The collection and use of data meet accepted ethical principles and pro-visions for confidentiality.	If an audit involves collecting information directly from patients, carers, or staff, care is taken to ensure that the procedure for collecting data and the information recorded are consistent with accepted ethical principles. Audit data are collected, handled, and presented consistent with agreed confidentiality policies related to audit.
	9	Data are analysed using appropriate methods.	The methods used for grouping data collected for an audit and the statistics used for analysis of the data provide a complete, accurate, and unbiased picture of actual practice.
	10	Data are presented to show clearly the relationship of actual practice to the objectives and to good practice.	The methods used for presenting data help the audit group members to understand how actual practice compares with good practice (as defined by the measures used in the audit) and whether or not objectives for the audit are being met.
EVALUATE	11	Formal evaluation of the data is carried out by the audit group to analyse the findings and to identify any shortcomings in the provision of care and their causes.	In the evaluation process, the members of the audit group: • Compare actual practice with good practice. • Analyse cases, occurrences, or situations which are not consistent with the audit measures and decide if the lack of consistency is or is not clinically acceptable. • Identify problems in the provision of care and their causes.
	12	Needed improvements in practice are identified by the audit group.	Improvements identified are related to the agreed audit objectives, reflect the audit group's analysis of causes of problems which are affecting care or services, and are consistent with recognized good practice.
ACT	13	An action strategy and an action implementation plan are developed to achieve needed improvements in practice.	Thge action strategy uses a variety of approaches, as needed, to achieve and maintain improvements. The action implementation plan includes: • Specific steps to be taken to address causes of problems identified and to achieve the needed improvements. • Individuals who are named as responsible to carry out the action. • Deadlines for execution of actions. • How and when the effectiveness and efficacy of the action is to be assessed.
	14	The action plan is implemented.	Evidence is available to confirm that audit findings have been acted upon or to support reasons for lack of action. Stakeholders in an audit are informed about action planned or taken as part of an audit.
REPEAT	15	Data collection, analysis, evaluation, and action are repeated as many times as required to confirm that improvements needed to meet the desired level of quality have been achieved and sustained.	Repeat data collection is designed to assess the effects of the action taken on the achievement of needed improvements. Several cycles of audit may be required to achieve the desired level of quality. When the decision is made not to reaudit, the reasons are stated clearly, for example, the needed improvements in care have been achieved.

Contact your local clinical audit department, your Primary Care Audit Group or Medical Audit Advisory Group, your professional organization, or the NCCA for more information on the NCCA Criteria for Clinical Audit.

13. Draft template of clinical audit report for a trust board

---

CLINICAL GOVERNANCE IN LONDON REGION

Draft template of clinical audit report for a Trust Board

Acknowledgements

The Regional Office would like to thank Dr Mark Charny, director of the National Centre for Clinical Audit and Sue Lydeard and colleagues at the Hammersmith Hospitals NHS Trust for their contributions to this template.

The audit programme

1. **Background**

   o Review of previous year's out-turn and how lessons learned have been applied in current year to which the report relates

2. **Selection of topics**

   How the audits carried out in the current year were chosen, including –

   o The driving force – bottom up, or top down?

   o The extent of involvement – i.e. multidisciplinary, uni-professional, multi-agency

   o Which groups were involved (local residents, patients, the Health Authority, local GP's/PCG's, the Trust Board, Clinicians of all professions in the Trust etc.)?

   o How were they involved?

   o What criteria were used to select the audits (e.g. national priorities such as

Calman/Hine, local priorities identified by the DPH's Annual Report, high risk areas of work, complaints, anomalous patterns of usage or outcomes or cost effectiveness, clinical interest, etc.)?

o How were the criteria applied ot assessed? Which group considered the inputs from stakeholders and how did they apply the criteria?

o Were any changes made to the original programme (planned audits not carried out and audits not planned, actually undertaken) and, if so, what and why?

o How did these changes affect the balance to the audit programme by speciality/directorate? Are some specialities/directorates not represented and if so, why?

3. **Monitoring the programme**

o What system(s) is/are used for tracking the audit programme and individual audits within it?

o Brief description of the relevant structures in the trust (lines of accountability, routine review mechanisms, methods of intervention when findings cause concern etc.)

o Outline of any serious or significant problem(s) identified through audit and remedial action taken.

o By directorate, did the programmes meet their objectives/performance indicators, e.g. a well balanced programme with a variety of audit projects, tackling numerous issues – user views, guideline use, clinical effectiveness?

4. **Costs**

o Overview of the costs of the programme, with breakdown into standard categories such as audit staff, computer equipment, software, licensing, training & travel, consumables, and clinical staff and non-staff time, where quantifiable.

o Were there any excessive costs per project, which do not demonstrate value for audit money, when comparing the value of the project to the delivery of patient care? Do changes need to be made to the programme for the following year to prevent this recurring?

5. **Critical Analysis**

o Highlights of any important areas of care, specialities, or professions not included in the audit programme, with reasons.

o Lists of audits undertaken during the year, with summary of impact on patient care. This can be a tabulated summary of the individual audits with totals of quantitative information, or a demonstration of impact via patient complaints/compliments system/focus groups.

    o What lessons have been learned from the approach taken to develop the audit programme (e.g. the timetable for planning, the choice of groups involved, the way in which the information is gathered and used, the balance of the programme?)

    o Links between the audit programme and other elements of clinical quality improvement such as risk management, clinical effectiveness programme, the complaints system etc.

6. **Recommendations for action**

    o Recommendations for action by the Trust Board and by others, such as the local Health Authority

    o Action plans developed, identifying actions to be taken, person responsible, progress reporting mechanism, dates for achievement.

Individual audits

For each audit (to be an annex of the programme report)

- **Title** – a brief title;
- **Participants** – a brief résumé of principal stakeholders, what approach was used to involve them, and in what aspects of the audit were they involved;
- **Standards** – the standards used to define the objective of the activity
    - o the source of these standards (benchmarking data, consensus statements, systematic reviews, national service frameworks, key literature etc);
- **Objectives** – an outline of the project objectives, providing a basis for measurement of the success of the audit versus resource use;
- **Methods** – a short description of methods (whose care was audited, what aspects of care were audited, by whom was the data collection undertaken, what audit method was used, what data were collected, which individuals or wards or Trusts etc were the subject of comparative analysis);
    - How were the data peer reviewed and by whom?
- **Findings** – What were the findings?
    - What conclusions were drawn from the findings?
    - Were objectives achieved, and if not, why not?
- **Action** – What action was planned to remedy any deficiencies discovered in care?

– What action is being taken to remedy any deficiencies discovered in care?

– What evidence is there that care has improved (with an estimate of how much the care has improved for how many patients of what type(s);

    o describe any problems encountered that audit participants could not solve (e.g. individuals or groups who would not, or could not, participate; changes to skill mix which could not be achieved; shortage of resources which could not be corrected etc);

    o Has the audit highlighted any related areas of care that might be the subject of future audits and, if so, why?

- **Costs** – What were the direct costs of the audit (breakdown by standard category staff, consumables etc)?

  – What were the indirect costs of the audit (estimates of audit and/or clinical staff time in data collection, data processing, data analysis, peer review, taking action, reviewing progress etc)?

- **Follow up** – What lessons have been learned about the process of audit itself for the future (were the right groups involved, could more cost-effective methods have been used etc)?

      o Are there plans to carry out further audits of the same aspects of care and, if so, why and when?

      o What steps have been taken to share the experience of the audit with others inside and outside the Trust? (e.g. by contributing to the national audit index, presentations at local and national events etc)

- **Recommendations** – Are there recommendations for action by the clinical directorate, the Trust Board and others e.g. Health Authority arising out of the audit?

Note: Where some of these steps have not yet been completed the report should indicate what steps are planned to complete the cycle

14. Clinical negligence scheme for trusts – risk management standards – summary of standards and features *National Health Service Litigation Authority, 1999*

Standard	
1. Board Clinical Risk Management Strategy	• There is a Board minute with date accepting the strategy • The strategy has been promulgated to all staff via handbooks and other information • The strategy is available to the public via publications, notice boards etc. • The strategy is available to local purchasers • The Trust can produce documentary evidence demonstrating that the Board's strategy is being implemented • The Trust can produce documentary evidence demonstrating that the Board's strategy is being implemented and is subject to continuing review
2. Executive Director and Clinical Risk	• An executive director has been appointed to be responsible for clinical risk management • The strategy makes clear the responsibility of the executive director for risk management
3. Clinical Risk Manager/Group	• One or more persons is charged with the responsibility for co-ordination of clinical risk activities • Post holder(s) is/are accountable to the executive director responsible for risk management
4. Clinical Incident Reporting System	• Policy/procedure on incident reporting is available in 10 per cent of directorates • Incident reporting form gathers significant data about the event (date, time, patient identifiers, outline of incident, staff involved) • Incident reporting form requires fact not opinion • The incident reporting form requires immediate reporting of unexpected death/serious injury • The incident reporting form or other records first aid for non-patients • The incident reporting form or other allows for notification of equipment failure • The incident reporting form allows 'near misses' to be recorded • Summarized incident reports are provided regularly to relevant bodies for review and action • The Trust has a policy on the relationship between incident reporting and disciplinary action • There is a process in place for detailed investigation of major clinical incidents • Clinically related events are being reported as they occur and before claims are made • There is evidence of management action arising from incident reporting • Implementation of incident reporting is operating in 25 per cent of directorates • The person receiving incident reports has written instructions on action to be taken • Incidents are graded for their degree of risk upon receipt of a form and guidance is given for this • In the interests of patient safety, openness and constructive criticism of clinical care is actively encouraged • Implementation of incident reporting is operating in all specialities • Incident reporting is part of induction training for all clinical staff
5. There is a policy for rapid follow-up of major clinical incidents	• The policy covers responsibility for management of the incident • The policy is explicit about responsibility for informing patient(s) and relative(s) • The policy covers record keeping about the incident

Section 5 continued	• The policy is explicit about individuals in the Trust who must be informed • The policy details which other interested parties need to be informed of the event, e.g. GPs, purchasers, Community Health Council • The policy makes it explicit that patients must be notified before the media • The policy covers media relations and who will be responsible for them • For serial incidents there is a strategy for dealing with multiple enquiries
6. Managing complaints	• The method of dealing with complaints is clear and meets NHSE guidelines • Examples of up to five changes which reduce risk as a consequence of complaints can be demonstrated
7. Information on the risks and benefits of proposed treatment or investigation	• There is patient information available showing the risks/benefits of up to 20 common elective treatments • All consent forms used comply with NHSE guidelines for design and use • There is policy/guideline stating that consent for elective procedures is to be obtained by a person capable of performing the procedure • There is a clear mechanism for patients to obtain additional information about their condition • The consent policy is audited for compliance
8. Standards, use, storage and retrieval of medical records	• There is a unified medical record which all specialities use • Records are bound and stored so that loss of documents and traces are minimized for inpatients and outpatients • The medical record contains clear instructions regarding the filing of documents • Operation notes and other key procedures are readily identifiable • CTG and other machine produced recordings are securely stored and mounted • There is a computer (or other efficient system) for identifying and retrieving X-rays • The storage arrangements allow retrieval on a 24 hour/7 day basis • There is clear evidence of clinical audit of record keeping standards in high-risk specialities within 12 months prior to the assessment • There is a mechanism for identifying records which must not be destroyed • A&E records are contained within the main record for patients who are subsequently admitted • Nursing, medical and other records (e.g. care plans) are filed together when the patient is discharged • There is a system for measuring efficiency in the recovery of records for inpatients and outpatients • The medical record contains a designated place for the recording of hypersensitivity reactions • A&E records should have a GP copy, which should be sent after each A&E episode • There is clear evidence of clinical audit of record keeping standards in at least 50 per cent of specialities within 12 months prior to the assessment • An author of an entry in a medical record is clearly and easily identifiable • There is clear evidence of clinical audit of record keeping standards in all specialities within 12 months prior to the assessment • There is a computer based PAS or HISS

9. Induction and training	• All clinical (including medical) staff attend a mandatory general introduction course on joining the Trust • All clinical staff attend a specific induction appropriate to the specialty in which they are working • The Trust has a policy requiring relevant clinical staff to be competent to perform basic life support and can demonstrate there is a system in place that fulfils the policy • There is a procedure for verifying the registration of clinical staff • Any person operating diagnostic or therapeutic equipment must have a sufficient understanding of its use to do so in a safe and effective manner • Training records of cardiopulmonary resuscitation training are kept • Clinical risk management is included in the general induction arrangements for all health care staff • The Trust has clear policies for addressing shortfalls in the conduct, performance and health of clinical staff • The Trust has an induction system covering all temporary (locum, bank or agency) clinical staff to ensure that such employees are competent to perform the duties of their post • Medical staff in training can demonstrate that they are technically competent to undertake their duties • The Trust has a clear policy requiring a consultant to have attended a relevant training programme before embarking on techniques which are new to him or her and which are not part of an ethical committee approved research programme • 90 per cent of eligible staff have attended cardiopulmonary resuscitation training in the last 12 months • There is a section on clinical risk management in the medical staff handbook incorporating policies and procedures
10. Clinical risk management system	• All clinical risk management standards and processes are in place and operational • A formal risk management forum exists where clinical risk issues are discussed • A risk management policy is implemented through the general management arrangements of the Trust • A Trust-wide clinical risk assessment has been conducted • There is evidence of implementation of recommendations made from the risk assessment
11. Clinical care	• All specialties have in place an integrated policy that identifies and addresses the needs of the patient prior to, and in preparation for, discharge from hospital • There are appropriate systems in place for the safe storage and administration of human blood and blood products • The Trust applies the advice of the National Confidential Enquiries • Clinical areas admitting emergencies are appropriately staffed at all times • There are clear lines of accountability and responsibility for staff working in another organization's facility • The Trust can demonstrate that there is a clear documented system of management and communication throughout all stages of patient care • Non-emergency surgery out of hours is reduced to a minimum • There are specific clinical standards for each specialty
12. Management and communication in maternity care	• The arrangements are clear concerning which professional is responsible for the patient's care at all times • The professional responsible for intra-partum care is clearly identified • There are referenced, evidence-based multidisciplinary policies for

Section 12 continued	the management of all key conditions/situations on the labour ward. These are subject to review at intervals of not more than 3 years. The following topics will be expected to be covered: diabetes; major haemoglobinopathy; severe hypertension; multiple pregnancy; breech presentation including version and selection for vaginal delivery; eclampsia; prolapsed cord; severe post-partum haemorrhage; ante-partum haemorrhage including placental abruption; shoulder dystocia; failed adult intubation; rupture of the uterus; unexplained intra-partum collapse (including amniotic fluid embolism); water birth; anatomical definition and repair of perineal tear; management of women who decline blood products; prophylactic antibiotics for Caesarean section; prostaglandins use; thrombo-prophylaxis in Caesarean section. • There is an agreed mechanism for direct referral to a consultant from a midwife • There is personal handover of care when medical or nursing shifts change • There is a clear documented system of management and communication throughout the key stages of maternity care • All clinicians should attend 6-monthly multidisciplinary in-service education/training sessions on the management of 'high risk' labours and CTG interpretations • There is a named consultant obstetrician and clinical midwife with designated responsibility for labour ward matters • There is clear guidance on the transfer of care in the intra-partum period • The labour ward has sufficient medical leadership and experience to provide a reasonable standard of care at all times; specifically: consultant supervision should be available for the labour ward for a minimum of 40 hours per week of scheduled sessions; a doctor of at least 3 years' experience in obstetrics (or consultant on call) should be available within 30 minutes; a doctor of at least 12 months' obstetrics experience should be resident on the labour ward at all times or available within 5 minutes; and an anaesthetist with at least 1 year's experience should be available within 10 minutes. • The delivery interval for Caesarean section for foetal distress is subject to an annual audited standard • There is personal handover to obstetric locums, either by the post holder or senior member of the team, and *vice versa* • Emergency Caesarean section can be undertaken rapidly and within a short enough period to eliminate unacceptable delay
13. Management of care in Trusts providing Mental Health and Learning Disability services	• All service users are assessed for the possibility of self-harm or harm to others (including suicide risk and assessment of risk of violence). The persons making the assessment are appropriately trained • Appropriate measures are in place to prevent the risk of self-harm or harm to others by service users • There is a multidisciplinary care programme approach – including an executive director nominated as CPA lead and a named CPA co-ordinator • Appropriate care programme approach documentation is use
14. There should be clear procedures for the management of clinical risk in Trusts providing ambulance services	• Records are made of patients who refuse treatment or travel to hospital • There is a policy on the recognition of death by paramedical staff and when to stop a resuscitation attempt • Patients suffering trauma or accident are transported to a location appropriate to their clinical needs

15. Template of audit of risk management – report for a trust board

The risk management system with the right culture

1. Has the right culture been nurtured?
   For staff – providing not blame and shame but a learning environment
   For patients – with staff who will listen, apologize and learn from mistakes
   For management – accepting fault when appropriate and offering timely and appropriate compensation

2. Has the right system been developed?
   What management arrangements are in place to involve staff, including senior clinicians, in processes such as the claims review committee?
   Is the risk management system devolved to the appropriate directorate level? Is the clinical director responsible for reducing risk in the directorate? At what level are data analysed?
   Are complaints linked to adverse incident reporting?
   Are adverse event data computerized?
   Is there a dedicated expert staff? Is the Trust getting smarter at analysing adverse events?

Current use of the system

Describe:

1. The number of significant adverse events
2. The number of claims substantiated, and damages paid
3. Training, how much and to whom
4. A synopsis of detailed investigations undertaken following serious or numerous adverse events
5. Trust performance relating to each CNST standard
6. The link between health and safety and risk management
7. Costs

Impact on patient care

1. Describe any new policies formulated as a result of major problems identified by the risk management system. For each new policy:
   What were the problems identified?
   What was the policy written?
   What management action was agreed?
   Have the original adverse events been reduced?
2. Provide a complaints analysis
3. Report any patient survey related to risk management

Value for money

Describe:

1. The budget for risk management
2. The contingency budget for claims
3. The costs of legal fees
4. The CNST costs
5. The comparative analysis with other similar Trusts when data available

Acknowledgements to David Stark, Alison Glover and Louise Boden from University College London Hospital and Jonathan Secker-Walker from Healthcare Resources Risk International. The NHS Executive, London Region (1999). Clinical governance in London Region, Draft template of audit risk management report for a Trust Board (http://www.doh.gov.uk/ntro/risktemp.htm).

Appendix 2
Glossary

Care pathway

A care pathway determines locally agreed, multidisciplinary practice based on guidelines and evidence where available, for a specific patient/client group. It forms all or part of the clinical record, documents the care given and facilitates the evaluation of outcomes for continuous quality improvement.

Clinical audit

The systematic and critical analysis of the quality of clinical care, including the procedures for the diagnosis, treatment and care, the associated use of resources and the resulting outcome and quality of life for the patient.

Clinical effectiveness

The extent to which clinical interventions maintain and improve health and secure the greatest possible health gain from available resources.

Clinical governance

A framework through which NHS organisations are accountable for continuously improving the quality of their services and safeguarding high standards of care by creating an environment in which clinical care will flourish.

Clinical supervision

A formal process of professional support and learning which enables individual practitioners to develop knowledge and competence, assume responsibility for their own practice and enhance consumer protection and safety of care in complex clinical situations.

Continuous professional development

'An individual taking responsibility for the development of his/her own career by systematically analysing development needs, identifying and using appropriate methods to meet these needs and regularly reviewing achievement compared against personal and career objectives.'

Controls assurance

The Cadbury report produced in 1992 recommended that the Board of Directors of each listed company registered in the United Kingdom should report on the effectiveness of the company's system of internal control. This recommendation applies to the public as well as the private sector. With respect to the NHS this means that the concept of 'controls assurance' requires that every Health Authority and Trust Board is satisfied that systems are in place within the organisation to ensure that risks are properly assessed and managed.

Corporate governance

The high standards of conduct expected of those who work in the Health Service are based on the recognition that patients come first and on the accountability to Parliament (the Welsh Assembly, the Scottish Parliament and the Northern Ireland Office for Wales, Scotland and Northern Ireland respectively) and to taxpayers on the effective use of public funds.

Cost benefit

The cost benefit of a service is determined by the absolute benefit of various models of care and is considered to be the gold standard of economic analysis. All the benefits (direct, indirect and intangible) are valued in the same units as the costs of interventions or treatments.

Cost effectiveness

The cost effectiveness of a particular form of health care depends upon the ratio of the costs of health care to its health outcomes.

Cost minimisation

Cost minimisation is a method used for comparing the costs of two similar interventions which have, for a particular condition, an equal outcome.

Cost utility

This method allows comparison between the relative efficiency of health care interventions for different conditions and uses a combination of mortality and morbidity data into a single measure. A typical example is the use of the Quality Adjusted Life Year (QUALY). This method can be used to compare different treatments.

Electronic Health Record (EHR)

This describes the health care of a person from cradle to grave in all settings including the outcomes of the periodic episodes of care held in the EPR.

Electronic Patient Record (EPR)

This describes the episode of care provided by mainly one organisation, e.g. a period of time spent in hospital for a total hip replacement, or in a specialist unit or mental health NHS trust.

Evidence-based medicine

The process of systematically reviewing, appraising and using contemporaneous research findings as the basis for clinical decisions.

Evidence-based health care

The means by which current best evidence from research can be judiciously and conscientiously applied in the prevention, detection and care of health disorders.

Evidence-based management

The application of the research evidence to needs assessment, planning, commissioning and other management processes.

Guidelines

Systematically developed statements to assist practitioner and patient decisions about appropriate health care for specific clinical circumstances.

Health outcomes

The attributable effect of intervention or its lack on a previous health state.

Independent Complaints Advocacy Services (ICAS)

These services provide independent support to people who want to complain and complement existing advocacy services.

Lifelong learning

All health care staff should have the up to date skills and knowledge required to deliver high quality care through continuous learning and training.

National Service Frameworks

National Service Frameworks define service models for a specific service or care group by bringing together the best evidence of clinical and cost effectiveness with the views of service users to determine the best ways of providing particular services.

Mentoring

A supportive nurturing relationship which provides inspiration and help by a mentor to a mentee to enhance the latter's skills and confidence.

Peer review

An assessment of the quality of care provided by a clinical team with a view to improving patient care.

Patient Advice and Liaison Services (PALS)

Patient Advice and Liaison Services provide 'on-site' help to patients within NHS trusts. Their role is to provide information to patients about health and health services locally including voluntary organisations and support groups. PALS play a key role in resolving concerns and problems quickly before they become serious and put patients in touch with specialist independent advocacy services if they wish to complain formally.

Patients' Forum

A Patients' Forum is a statutory body made up of patients and others from the local community and has powers to inspect all aspects of the work of trusts, general practice, NHS work carried out in the independent sector and wider health issues.

Risk management

A means of reducing the risks of adverse events occurring in organisations by systematically assessing, reviewing and then seeking ways to prevent their occurrence. Clinical risk management takes place in a clinical setting.

The seven pillars of clinical governance

Clinical governance has been further refined into the 'seven pillars' which are:

- clinical effectiveness
- risk management
- research and development

- use of the workforce
- training and education
- use of information
- patient/user feedback

The Commission for Health Improvement (CHI)

A statutory body whose function is to support the development of high quality clinical practice consistently across the NHS. Its role is to provide national leadership on the principles of clinical governance and to support those organisations which are having difficulty setting up clinical governance arrangements locally when usual channels have failed.

The Commission for Healthcare Audit and Inspection (CHAI)

This is the successor to the Commission for Health Improvement. Its role has been widened from the original remit of CHI to cover inspection of the health service and the private sector, the production of performance indicators and trust NHS performance ratings, an annual report to parliament on the state of the NHS, value for money audits and the work of the Mental Health Act Commission.

The Commission for Patient and Public Involvement in Health (CPPIH)

This body is responsible for making appointments to Patients' Forums and complements existing patient organisations. It sets national standards, provides training and monitoring of PALS, Patients' Forums and the Independent Complaints Advocacy Services (ICAS). At the community level, the CPPIH operates through 'local networks' which facilitate the involvement of local groups in feedback on health services development and provision. Local networks also commission the ICAS for patients, carers or families who need independent support in making a complaint.

The National Clinical Assessment Authority (NCAA)

The NCAA provides a support service to the NHS when the performance of an individual doctor causes great concern. The Authority provides advice, takes referrals and carries out targeted assessments where necessary. The Authority currently serves all NHS doctors working in England only and doctors working for the prison service.

The National Patient Safety Agency (NPSA)

The NPSA is a Special Health Authority which co-ordinates the efforts of the staff in the NHS to report and learn from adverse events in the health service.

The Modernisation Agency

The Modernisation Agency is a part of the Department of Health whose role is to help health care staff redesign local health services in accordance with good practice.

The National Electronic Library for Health

This is a virtual library for health professionals. Its role is to provide easy access to the research papers and reviews on best current knowledge about health problems, their causes, prevention and treatment.

The National Institute for Clinical Excellence (NICE)

A statutory body which provides national evidence-based clinical guidelines for local adaptation, clinical audit methodologies and information on good practice. It covers the English and Welsh NHS. The Clinical Standards Board carries out a similar function in Scotland and, at the time of writing, Northern Ireland is still consulting about its structures.

The NHSnet

The secure national network developed exclusively for the NHS for conveying electronic information.

The NHS Performance Assessment Framework

This is the mechanism for Health Authorities and PCGs to use to help them monitor the delivery of health services against the plans for improvement. It identifies six main areas in which performance can be measured.

The NHS Performance Ratings

A system of measures to help the public assess the performance of NHS organisations - also known as the 'star ratings'.

The NHS University (NHSU)

The role of the NHSU is to ensure that NHS staff continue to have access to high quality education and training. The NHSU is a real bricks and mortar institution and a virtual body. It plays an important role in ensuring that the learning and development needs of NHS staff are covered and are linked to the strategic direction of the NHS Plan.

Appendix 3
Useful websites

NHS UK - gateway to National Health Service organisations on the Internet
  www.nhs.uk

Commission for Health Improvement
  www.chi.nhs.uk

National Institute for Clinical Excellence
  www.nice.org.uk

The Modernisation Agency
  www.nhs.uk/modernnhs

Scottish Intercollegiate Guidelines Network
  pc47.cee.hw.ac.uk/sign/home.htm

National Electronic Library for Health
  www.nelh.nhs.uk

Clinical Governance website
  www.doh.gov.uk/clinicalgovernance/index.htm

Primary Care National Electronic Library for Health
  www.nelh-pc.nhs.uk

NHS Clinical Governance Support Team
  www.cgsupport.org

National Patient Safety Agency
  www.npsa.org.uk

Clinical Standards Board for Scotland
  www.clinicalstandards.org

Research Findings Electronic Register (ReFeR)
www.doh.gov.uk/research

Register of Controlled Trials
www.controlled-trials.com

National Primary Care Research and Development Centre, University of Manchester
www.npcrdc.man.ac.uk

The Cochrane Library, Cochrane Collaboration, Oxford
www.update-software.com/cochrane/ - database on disk and CD-Rom
Update software issued quarterly

Effective Healthcare Bulletins, University of York
www.york.ac.uk/inst/crd

Bandolier
www.jr2.ox.ac.uk/Bandolier

Critical Appraisal Skills Programme (CASP)
www.ihs.ox.ac.uk/casp

National Prescribing Centre
www.npc.co.uk

York Centre for Reviews and Dissemination
www.york.ac.uk/inst/crd/sites.htm

The Electronic Library for Social Care
www.elsc.org.uk

The National Clinical Assessment Authority
www.ncaa.nhs.uk

NHS Beacons
www.nhs.uk/beacons

NHS Performance Ratings
www.doh.gov.uk/performanceratings

Clinical Evidence
www.clinicalevidence.org

Workforce Development Confederations
www.wdconfeds.org

NHS Direct Online
www.nhsdirect.nhs.uk

Human Rights Act 1998
www.doh.gov.uk/humanrights

Information on Consent Procedures
www.doh.gov.uk/consent

Resuscitation Council (UK)
www.resus.org.uk/pages/dnar.htm

NHS University
www.nhsu.nhs.uk

Involving Patients
www.doh.gov.uk/involvingpatients

NHS Litigation Authority
www.nhsla.com

Index

All references to diagrams, tables and any other non-textual material are in italics.